Carol
Rata, Rata, Rata

Rose Lamatt

Also by Rose Lamatt

Just a Word

Is Life One Big Goodbye

Connected

Voiceless Cry

Acknowledgements

Thank you Carol, for being my friend

Prologue

I stopped at the post office to pick up my mail. Bending down, putting the key in the PO Box, I looked up and saw Carol. At least she looked like Carol. Tall, long legs, brown hair, even her clothing were Carol's: light blue four button shirt, pink paisley slacks, even her shoes Carol's—loafers.

I stared at her, not realizing how long, and when she turned to look at me; her eyes were Carol's, soft, round brown eyes. The woman smiled, Carol's smile.

Finally I opened my mouth, "I'm sorry for staring, but you look just like someone I used to know."

"Oh, people tell me that all the time."

"No, really, you could pass for her twin."

"Is she nice?" the woman asked.

"Yes, she was very nice. She passed away."

"Oh, I'm sorry."

"That's okay. Thank you for bringing her back to me. I can't believe the likeness. Please excuse me for staring so long. I hope you have a nice day." And Rose walked fast out of the Post Office, thinking, she'd seen a ghost.

In an unsettled state of mind she decided a movie would be just what she needed. Be out, around others, she thought, and get rid of the ghost she saw.

Most days she stayed inside, working on the computer, or reading a book. She didn't do much of anything anymore, except see doctors, grocery shop, and a movie, once in a while. She'd even quit going to church on Sunday. Without church on Sunday she had no reference day. One day blended into others. At times, she'd wake on Monday, thinking it was Friday, finding she had another week to get through.

Now she headed to the next town, thinking, she'd see something funny, not a mystery, no killing, that's for sure. She wasn't fond of murder pictures, especially ones that showed blood and guts. Although she liked old Alfred Hitchcock shows from years ago, now being shown around dinner time. She didn't stay up late anymore, like in days of Jonny Carson's tonight show. No, she usually went to bed around nine with a book, then found the book on her chest an hour later. She then turned out the light, said her Rosary, falling asleep without ever getting through all the beads.

But now the theater took her away from herself and on to the screen. She watched a family go through raising two children, girl and boy. Puberty came and Father tried telling the boy what will happen to his body, and Mom told daughter what will happen to her body. But it seemed both children had learned this from school friends. The movie audience broke out in laughter, along with Rose.

Walking out of the theater, still a smile on her face, a stranger remarked, "Wasn't that the funniest movie you ever saw?"

"Yes, I loved it. Especially when the dog jumped out the window..." Rose answered.

Still smiling, she made it to her car, happy ... just to be.

In the car, back to reality, she thought, *grocery store? I do need something for dinner.*

Light headed, from only a small bag of popcorn and no lunch, she walked the isles searching for dinner. She settled on already roasted chicken. Go home, eat while watching television, day over. Or would she want to go out again tomorrow? No.

Maybe she'd get carrots, celery, and onions, make soup tomorrow, with the left overs. Make a miraqua, with a little wine thrown in, for sweetness. Her father taught her to cook, but she learned the word miraqua in eighth grade cooking class. She loved cooking, watched cooking shows on television. She'd come up with a meal that Carol and her had not had before, then either they'd love it or hate it, throwing out the whole mess and going out for burgers. Most meals were made with love back then. Now she ate, made it last another meal, and got it over with.

At the produce counter she picked through bags of grapes. *Why were they all old and rotten?* Something to do with the GMO, she guessed. What exactly did Genetically Modified Organism mean anyway?

Searching for potatoes that didn't have growth spurts, she bumped into the person standing next to her. "Oh, I'm sorry," she said, only to see Carol's lookalike again.

"How nice, we meet twice in one day," the paisley pants woman said.

"Yes. It must be an omen or something."

"I'm glad you have a smile on your face now, not like earlier, when I scared the beegeebers out of you."

"Yeah, I just came from a funny movie and highly recommend it." They talked awhile, Rose telling her about the movie. "See it, if you want a good laugh."

"I'll try, but right now I better get home and make dinner, before my husband disowns me." And the lookalike walked away.

She's nice, Rose thought, while waiting on the checkout line. Why didn't I get her name or where she lives? She ran back to produce hoping to see Carol's twin, get her name and number, but she couldn't find her anywhere.

Rose carried groceries up the stairs and couldn't get the woman out of her mind. Twice in one day, what are the odds?

She put milk, eggs and bread in the fridge. She'd take care of the rest after the bathroom visit.

Walking past the dining room table, her eyes caught hold of something that wasn't there before. A yellow sheet of paper and tan package sat in the middle of the table. She'd showered and had breakfast at this table. They weren't there before. She knew she was going through a difficult time in her life. She'd been going through a difficult time for quite a while now. It seemed the older she got the more confusing life became. But she knew one thing. The package and yellow paper were not there earlier. She was positive. Was she starting to question her own mind?

She unfolded the paper, beautiful cursive writing. Carol's script. How is it possible? She's been gone for years. Rose herself had put Carol's remains in the ocean, in front of the condo they had lived. She had watched a double rainbow develop after disposing the remains in the water. This couldn't be Carol's handwriting. She rubbed her forehead, confused and slightly disoriented and read:

My dearest beloved,

I know you are lost now, not taking care of me. I know you think of the times we had together, playing golf and soaking up the morning sun at the pool. You asked, so many times, how could I leave you after I got Alzheimer's. You tried your best to care for me and developed heart disease because of it. You came to visit me when you finally put me in a nursing home, as I asked you to do when first diagnosed. You came ten years visiting and talk to me. I couldn't speak after two years into the disease, but I always understood you. I was mad most of the time because you felt you needed to care for me, while I wanted you to go on with your life and be happy. You came with a smile on your face and sang to me while you fed me, even though I yelled in a voice you didn't understand. I was grateful you were there to pray for me. You prayed I wouldn't have the disease. You prayed and prayed for a misdiagnosis, or doctor's mistake, a vitamin deficiency, maybe.

I'm writing to tell you I am watching over you. I know at times that you feel me close and try to ignore me. But I persist until you take notice. When you get depressed, I am down with you. When you cry, I cry along with you. I want you to know you are never alone, that I am always with you, in good and bad. You might want to call me your angel. I don't know if I qualify at six-feet tall, as you remember me. But now I can be any size, even the ant that walks beside you on the sidewalk. When you sit on the porch and hear the birds, it's me singing to you. When you feel a breeze brush against your cheek, it's me blowing you a kiss. When you saw the double rainbow after you put my ashes in the ocean, it was you and I, always together, till eternity.

I have learned a lot about this other place called heaven. You can go anywhere you want, and 'The Boss' doesn't yell if you do something wrong. He says, there is no wrong. Everyone is nice. I play golf whenever I want, and can be with you at the same time. You see Rose there is no time or space in heaven. Think of it as a body made up of millions of cells, one cell plays golf, while another cell does something else. Everyone loves one another, like you and I did, when I was with you in body. We lived a heaven on earth, Rose. Remember when we moved to Florida, we were going to change the world by smiling at everyone we passed on the sidewalk. I think we did change lives. One person here you would remember. The homeless woman we treated to breakfast? She's here. She's thanked me and told me to thank you. If it wasn't for us that morning buying her breakfast, she would have never changed her life around, found a job and got off drugs. So you see dearest one, we did change the world. Now take these pages I left you and make another book. Tell everyone what it's like to have Alzheimer's/Dementia, living in a facility or anywhere.

The phone rang. The caller telling Rose she'd won a trip to the Bahamas. "When?" she asked, "Where in the Bahamas?" They didn't answer and repeated saying she'd won a trip to the Bahamas. Rose asked another question, then realized it was a robot recording, like so many received in prior years, and she hung up.

She went back reading.

So you see we can change the world. I'll be leaving you little notes in the future to let you know I haven't left you alone. I am always at your side.

Till next time, take good care of yourself, dear one.

Carol

Rose sat staring at the yellow paper. Twice in one day—the lookalike twin, and now this.

She had longed for this, so why didn't she believe? She'd seen butterflies come, almost kiss her cheek. She'd heard red birds sing, follow her, even in cement parking lots. She knew deep down they were signs. Something said so. So why didn't she believe it? The double rainbow that came after putting Carol's ashes in the ocean, should have told her something was happening. Now, Carol's hand writing on the yellow legal paper she always used. How much proof did she need?

She sat on the bed, staring at the paper, rubbing it between her fingers, reading again and again. Was she losing it or had she already lost it? Finally she opened the tan package finding more written pages. She caressed the gold 'rose' around her neck. The one she'd given Carol for her birthday,

Valentine's Day, long ago, then later took the rose back when Carol got ill. She began reading.

Chapter 1

How do I say what's happening, when I can't speak words taught by my mother and father. Do I say it in my voice? If I did you wouldn't understand. Only those with Alzheimer's understand. Maybe I'll ask someone to write it. Maybe I can ask with my eyes? That's all I have left to communicate. I could use my hands and hit you, but that would make you angry. No, I'll communicate with my eyes.

***

At the dining table in the nursing home I'm seated with three others. Millie, who is like me because we understand each other … speak the same language, *our* words. Not like nurses or aides who care for us. They speak Rose's words. I understand *their* words but they don't understand *mine*. Not sure why. It's like the world has turned upside down and I don't know which is right, mine or theirs.

Even though the doctor diagnosed me with Alzheimer's, I know I don't have it. I hear others speak my language and they have the same illness. The doctors were wrong. People are made to believe their loved one has Alzheimer's, when they don't. We know the answer, but no one's asking us.

Millie asks, when am I'm going to eat. "Sha, sha, sha," I tell her. *I don't know.*

Millie's tray sits in front of her but she can't pick up the fork, her hands don't work. The aide brings my tray: mashed potatoes, green beans, ground turkey with gravy, apple pie for desert, and a carton of milk. I look at the food, then scoop a spoon full of mashed potatoes in the empty plastic glass. I add gravy and pie. *Is that right?* It looks okay, but the man opposite me looks mad. Doesn't he know this is the way I eat? Another lady sits with us. She sleeps in a wheel-chair-bed contraption, her head tilted up and her legs out in front of her. She seems happy, that's important. With a plastic spoon I stir my food. *Why does that man keep staring at me?* We ate breakfast at eight o'clock this morning, but I didn't get a chance to finish. They cleared us out of the dining room, yelling, "C'mon we have activities, and need the room. We have to leave the dining room, Now!"

It's twelve-thirty now and I know they'll make us leave at one o'clock. An aide puts a straw in the milk carton and holds it to my lips. "Sha, sha, sha," I say, *thank you.* But she goes on doing what she's doing and doesn't acknowledge. The milk is good, I'm thirsty, and God knows when she'll be back.

Someone drops a fork on the floor and starts yelling. It disturbs me, and others. We speak our language, the one we understand. *Why doesn't someone pick it up, and help the person who dropped it?* Everyone agrees.

Someone decides to run out the door. An aide grabs hold of her, "Sally, get back in your chair and finish your lunch." Sally mumbles something, but I'm too far away to hear exact words. Knowing Sally, she probably said, *Leave me the hell alone.* I've learned in a short time, Sally doesn't get mad often, but when she does, watch out. This is why the room's in mass confusion; they know Sally throws things when she's really mad. People run all over the place, yelling. It's awful. Don't they understand, I want to finish my lunch? Then I can walk the halls.

Finally, I get a spoonful of makings in my mouth. It's sweet, the pie I guess. I like sweets. Again that guy watches me. I turn to Millie and ask, Sha, sha, sha, sha? *Why is he staring at me?* He watches everyone, she says, it just happens to be you today. Just when Millie gets her words out an aide moves her. I yell at the aide, "Rata, Rata, Rata" *She hasn't finished her meal.* But the aide doesn't listen. I feel sorry for Millie. I go back working on mashed potatoes and apple pie. I wish these utensils were easier to use. I lean down grab hold of the straw and sip milk, it helps the potatoes go down, but I wish the guy would stop looking at me. His glasses fall low on his nose, and all I see are the whites of his eyes. They're large, glaring. Finally, the aide undoes the brakes on his chair.

"You're next Carol," she says, wheeling him out.

"Rata, Rata, Rata." *Oh, no, I'm not done with my lunch.* She doesn't hear me. I stuff another spoonful in my mouth, I'm so hungry. Then I see the big-fat aide head my way. Oh no, not her. She hurts me. Then I hear, "C'mon Carol, let's go to the bathroom, and then to activities. They're having a piano player today. You'll enjoy him."

Enjoy him? I want to eat! I'm hungry! Doesn't she get it? All she needs to do is look at my plate. I haven't finished. She grabs me, hard, under the arm, pinching skin. *Dammit!* I'll have more bruises tomorrow. She pulls me. I stay seated. But she's three times larger than me and isn't nice. She pulls me up again, this time right out of the chair. Sometimes my legs don't listen and do what they want. She pulls me down the hall. I'm scared. She's hurting me. "Come, Carol, we're going to wash our hands and face, and go to the bathroom."

Holding back I follow, but she's bigger and stronger and hurts my wrist. I swing at her with my free hand, and miss. "You're not going to hit me, now, are you, Carol?" she says.

Wrong thing to do.

In the bathroom she pulls my pants down, undoes the brief and shoves me on the toilet. I get up. She pushes me down—hard. "Rata, Rata, Rata,

Rata." I say, and stay seated. She slams a wet cloth onto my face. *It's cold,* and I tinkle at the same time.

"Good girl," she says. "You went potty." As if I'm five years old. I'm no child. I know what I'm doing.

Pulling me off the toilet she puts another brief on and pulls up my pants, tucking in my shirt. Why is she so rough? Rose was never rough with me. Rose sat on the bathroom floor and sang to me, when I had to go potty. She was kind. But this aide needs schooling on how to treat a person.

Finally done, I make my rounds down the hall. I meet Sally, Marti, John, and Josephine. They're nice. Sally tells us why she had to leave the dining room. She had a feeling someone was in her room stealing things. *Did they?* we ask. She says, *No, I was wrong. But I felt it.* We talk to each other wondering why others don't understand us. *We have our own club*, we agree. *Others speak Spanish, and we don't understand them. There's no difference, we have our language,* Sally says. *I know someone was in my room messing with my stuff. I just know it.*

Sally thinks she can read minds, and I'm not sure she can't. We all have a little of that in us.

Marti says, *Come in my room. I'll show you pictures of my family.* We look at pictures and he explains who everyone is. His brother looks just like him. Although, he says, *My father was a mean ole sonabitch.* We look through clothes in his closet and he offers me a shirt. *Thank you Marti,* I say, in our voice, and leave. I get lost along the way and wind up in someone's room. Tired, I lie on the bed and fall asleep.

Chapter 2

Why can't they leave me alone? Let me be. It's always, do this, do that. You need to eat, you need to wash, you need to dress, and you need to pee. You need, you need, you need, every day it's the same. Why can't they just leave me alone? I don't hurt them. Why do they give *me* pain?

Rose left me here and hasn't come back. I wonder if I'll ever see her again. I don't understand what happened. We were home, doing fine, until she wanted me clean all the time. My hair washed, my teeth brushed, my face washed, take a shower, eat, go to the bathroom. Kind of the way I'm living now. Why did I have to wash so much?

While showering I threw her against the shower doors and ran to my bedroom. I didn't need a shower, we weren't going anywhere. What difference did it make? I didn't play outside in the dirt. I was in the house all day. How dirty could I be?

That last day, the spray hit my body feeling like stinging bees on my legs and feet. I had to get away before it hit my face, my eyes. Rose didn't listen. I told her, "Rata, Rata, Rata, Rata." Why didn't she understand, it hurt? I didn't mean to slam her against the doors. I had to. I had to get away.

I ran to my bedroom to be with my other friend, the one in the reflection box. She's nice, and has followed me here. She has dark brown hair, like me; brown eyes, like me. And she's tall, like me. She doesn't make me eat, dress and wash all the time. She doesn't tell me what to do. She smiles most of the time, except when she's mad, and then we're both mad.

The day of the shower, Rose followed me, bringing towels and cookies. I like cookies, chocolate chip my favorite. She pushed down on my shoulders, and I sat on the bed, as she wanted. I ate a cookie while she dried moisture from my body. Then she dressed me. Putting my sneakers on, I brought my leg up too high, and that's when it happened. I hit her with my knee, knocking her glasses off. She ran, yelling, her hand over her eye. I hurt her, I thought. I didn't mean to. Afraid, I sat on the bed eating my cookie. When she came back, she tried putting on my sneakers again. I wasn't about to lift my foot again and hurt her. So I just chomped on my cookie.

"Please Carol, lift your foot," she said.

But I didn't.

She got mad, and slapped me across the arm yelling, "Do it yourself!"

Well, what did she think? If I wanted to get dressed, I would. I didn't want to. I wanted to stay as

I was. *Leave Me Be*, I yelled in my voice, but she didn't hear. She never heard. She left for her bathroom, as always, and I ate my cookies in peace.

Later, cookies finished, I walked into the living room and overheard Rose on the kitchen phone, "I can't take it anymore." She cried to someone, "I just can't take it."

She can't take what? I felt sorry for her, apparently there was something bothering her, but I couldn't do anything about it.

Next she's pushing me out the door and into the car. *I don't want to go*, I said in my voice. I clung to the car door saying, *No, I don't want to go*, but she didn't hear, or didn't want to. Most of the time she acts like she doesn't understand me, which I don't get, because we always understood each another. We always got along. What happened? I noticed something different after the doctor called. What did he say?

Oh yes, we were staying at a motel on Long Island. We had taken the train from Florida to New York, and then rented a car, and Rose drove us to the motel. I remember sitting by the window reading the newspaper, sun shining bright, making lines across the rug. What was it the doctor said? Oh yes, "I'm sorry to tell you, but Carol has a dementia known as Alzheimer's", yes, that was it.

A few years later she stopped understanding me. I remember I had trouble putting words into sentences, and left coffee cups where they didn't belong, like in my bedroom closet or in the bathroom.

Not that I wanted to, I just forgot. Rose would find them later and bring them to me. Another time I ate a bunch of bananas, and she had a fit, saying I was going to have a stomach ache. I didn't. I just wanted something sweet. Often the phone rang and I knew who it was, but sometimes I didn't. "Carol, it's your friend, Jane," Rose said. Who the heck was Jane? I didn't know a Jane. Rose said we had played golf with her in a tournament a year ago. Well how the heck did she expect me to remember what I did a year ago? Maybe Rose met her, but I didn't. Anyway, that's when we started disconnecting, not able to understand one another. Was I confused? Or was it Rose? I stopped doing all investments. She handled everything: mortgage payments, condo bills, health insurance, and other household items. I wanted to handle things but they weren't in my language.

When we went to church I opened my hand, like Rose told me, and the priest put something in the palm of my hand. I kept it hidden from everyone until we got in the car and that's when I opened my hand and showed Rose. She got all bent out of shape and kept asking, "Why did you do that? Why didn't you put it in your mouth in church?"

Questions…questions…questions. I looked at the round disk in my hand. What was I supposed to do with it? "Put your tongue out," Rose said. I did. And she put the disk on my tongue then said, "Now eat it." I did. It tasted flat, not sweet. Tasted like cardboard. She then made a cross sign on my forehead, saying, "God, please forgive Carol." Then she said, "How could you keep the Host in your hand?"

After that everything was downhill. We'd play golf, and I'd forget where I hit the ball. We'd look for the ball while the foursome behind us got mad, waiting. Rose called them ahead of us, and when we found my ball it began all over again. Hole after hole I lost my ball, and hole after hole we let golfers behind go ahead. We stopped riding bikes when I rode too fast for Rose. Swimming was the only sport that lasted. I liked the pool, walking in the water and swimming laps. But after a while Rose had to say, stop, and help me up the pool steps out of the water. Our after dinner walks also stopped. I guess because I walked faster and longer than Rose. We'd been exercising years, staying healthy. Hours spent at the pool, beach, and golf course. But everything stopped.

Why? Was Rose sick?

***

The day after the shower door incident, she pushed and pulled wanting me in the car. But I held the door tight, with both hands. She said, "You're going on vacation. You'll like it. They have good food, and you can help lots of people."

I liked that. I am good at helping people. I've done it most of my life.

I let go of the door.

While riding, trees flew by faster and faster. She's driving too fast. "Rata, Rata, Rata, Rata," I said. "Rata, Rata, telling her *slow down*. But she didn't listen. I hadn't driven in a while, but I never drove this fast. She told me I couldn't drive anymore, afraid of an accident. Something to do with that 'A' word, and if I were in an accident I'd lose everything: condo, money, everything. I stopped when my accountant-advisor told me the same.

As she drove, I saw cars and people on the street, wondering, were they going to the same place, to help others?

An hour later she pulled into a parking space and got out. She came around my side and opened the door. I held onto the seat. *I can't get out.*

"C'mon Ca," she said. She called me 'Ca' most of the time, short for Carol. I liked Ca. I guess because Carol sounded so serious. Like, "Carol you have to wash your hair." Or "Carol you need to be careful."

She picked up my right leg, lifted it out of the car, then my other leg. She held my hands pulling me up. *She wants me with her,* I thought. She held my hands walking up the sidewalk toward the large brick building, four, five, stories high. Tall, no matter how you look at it. I didn't want to go, but I did, for her.

Inside I saw a lot of people in wheelchairs, some not. *I'll help the woman over there, she can't move.* The wheels of her chair were stuck against the wall. I tried breaking loose from Rose's hand. "No Carol, stay with me," she said. I thought, *this must be serious.*

"Rata, Rata, Rata," *I don't want to*, in my language, but she didn't understand. *I need to help the woman over there. Can't you see? She can't move her wheelchair. She wants to go somewhere.* Finally I broke loose. Rose came after me, but I'm fast. I heard the woman in the dark blue suit say, "Let her go, Rose. The aides will watch her."

I made it to the wheelchair woman, and asked where she wanted to go. She pointed down the hall, so I pushed. She's big and fat, but I'm strong. I can do it. Then I saw a man putting on his sweater. He had his arm where his head should go. Helping him, I undid the mess. Then I saw someone else. So many people need help. Rose was right. I *can* assist.

Later, Rose took me to a room. "This is *your* room, Carol. How do you like it?" She sounded serious again.

Looking around, I thought, nice, but nothing to write home about. Blue drapes on a window, a bed, dresser, chair and private bath … I won't need that. Rose said how nice the room was, "Don't you just love the colors?" she asked. Blue *is* my favorite color, so the drapes are nice. She says I'll like it while I'm here. But I wanted to walk, see who needed help. She told me I was coming to help. *Let me go help.*

Rose put clothes in dresser drawers and hung others in the closet. I started walking. "Wait," she said, but I was out the door before she could catch me. She never lets me do what I want. Always told me "No".

Where is she?

Chapter 3

Rose misses Carol and wants to visit her, but she's been told not to. "Carol needs to forget living with you and get used to living at the nursing home," they said.

It doesn't make sense. Why would they want me to just leave her and not visit? She'll forget me. I know she will. Especially having Alzheimer's, the forgetful disease.

Rose doesn't know what to do without Carol. Everything was done with Carol or with Carol in mind. How can she forget her?

They lost friends because friends didn't understand Alzheimer's. They didn't understand how a person changes. How they can become combative and lose the ability to talk in conversation. Friends didn't understand, but neither did Rose. But she knew Carol, and loved her.

The nursing home wants Rose to leave Carol there, as if she doesn't exist. She worries about her. What is she doing? Who is she talking to? Is she lonely? Is she pacing the halls as she paced at home? Is she eating? Rose left her at the nursing home. She's no different than the friends who forgot about her. And all because of one Word.

Chapter 4

Rose still hasn't come. I'm so tired, but I can't sleep. I need to find a way out of here. I want to go home.

Rose understands. She's seen me look at pictures of Mom and Dad and knows how much I miss them. I have to find them. I must find a way out of this maze. Why did she leave me here? Is she ill? I could take care of her.

I woke shaky this morning. My hands couldn't hold the comb when I combed my hair. Was it the new room? This blue room that Rose liked so much. Why did she leave me here? I know she said I was going to help people, but I could've done that during the day instead of sleeping here. I don't like new beds, new rooms, new anything. It's hard to get adjusted to 'new'. I like old, as in home.

Standing looking at my friend in the mirror I felt a little better. She also looked undone, unkempt, out-of-it, for a better word.

The building is so big. I have the feeling I'm in a hospital. I'd been in the hospital a few times, the last for lymph gland removal under my arm pits. All because of melanoma, the size of a dime, on my arm. I'd had it a year, but then the doctor said he didn't like the looks of it, and next thing I knew I had a six inch scar. Oh, it hurt. I remember crying when Rose came after the operation. "Why does it hurt so much?" I asked, but she couldn't answer. Maybe she was upset. I never thought about her being upset. I wonder if she's upset now.

I hear the door open and a woman dressed in a blue aide's uniform asks would I like breakfast. "Sha," I say. *Sure*, and touch her badge. *Vivian*.

"My name is Vivian. I'm happy to meet you Carol, and be of service."

That's a nice name. I don't think I ever knew a Vivian.

She combs the hairs out of place on my head. She's nice and I can use her help being I don't know where anything is.

"Do you need to use the bathroom before we go to breakfast?" she asks.

"Sha," *No*, I answer, along with shaking my head.

"Well then, we're ready for breakfast," and takes my hand, kind of the way Rose did.

We walk the long hall around holes. She tells me not to be afraid, everything is going to be all right. I'm not sure I believe that.

***

I walk the green hall after being taken out of the dining room from unfinished breakfast. *Why?* Because they just wanted us out of the dining room.

Why are there so many holes in the floor? They must be fixing it. I step from green tile to green tile, over the black holes. Who was so stupid to leave gaping holes in the floor? Why aren't barricades around them so we don't fall in? I jump my way around holes to the piano sound.

The mustache beret man is playing my favorite song, 'Oh we ain't got a barrel of money, maybe we're ragged and funny, but we travel along singing a song, side by side.'

I join others, "Rata, rata rata, rata, raaata," I can't sing like him. I like my words better. Rose and I sang it every year traveling to New York and back to Florida. She said it made the trip go faster. *It did.*

Well, enough of that.

I walk, hopping over holes. Someone's going to fall in if they're not careful. Not me, I have long legs and hop over them.

Ah, the Exit. Maybe I can get out there.

I hurry to the Exit sign, push the door. Darn, broken. I go up the hall and down the other, stepping over holes. I find another door, also broken.

Then see different doors, glass. I push. They open.

Oh, this is nice: green plants, flowers in pots and hanging baskets. I pull one basket toward me and smell the flowers, nice. Brown striped chairs and lounges line the patio. Kind of like what Rose and I had.

I've never been here. At the end of the patio I see an iron gate. I'll get out there. I push the gate, it won't open. *Um* ... low, I can climb over. One leg, then the other, good thing I'm tall. I'm over and finally outside.

Where's the ground? I walk around the round metal container. *Where's the ground?* Must be like the hall floor, they're working on it. Big holes.

"Carol. NO! Come ... Back ... Here. NOW!" Someone yells, running toward me. "Carol. Stop. Stay still!"

She latches onto my arm and pulls me back. "No, Carol," and lifts my leg onto cement. "Rata, Rata, Rata." *Let me go.* She pulls me inside the gate. I look back to where I was almost out of here. I'll come back another time when no one's around.

"Do you believe she climbed onto the other roof?" the aide tells another. "I almost lost her off the balcony. That would have made the papers. 'Woman steps off third floor balcony and breaks neck.' We'd surely be out of jobs."

She gives me juice and sets me in the activities room where people sit in chairs with large wheels. I drink juice while piano-man plays. I talk to Josephine, seated next to me. She tells me her son put her here because she was a bother to him. Was I a bother to Rose? Is that why I'm here? No, that can't be. It must be because Rose is ill. She told me I came here to help people. Finishing our juice I take our cups and throw them under the couch. *Bye*, Josephine says when a woman pushes her chair down the hall. Where's she going? Maybe she's getting out of here?

I get up and follow, remembering to step over holes. For some reason, chair wheels glide over the holes. I follow, leaving enough distance between us so the woman won't see me. I follow them into a room.

"Carol, you have to leave now," the woman says. I look at her, and back into the hall. When she leaves I go in and tuck Josephine in bed, nice and tight. She'll be warm and comfy now. I hear her snore. Like Rose said, "You're going to help people." I leave, making my way down the hall.

Chapter 5

Today I went on a small bus with other women. It was nice being outside and with others. Sally and Josephine went along and others I didn't know.

When we were dropped off a worker took us to a room where other women sat watching television. I said goodbye to Sally and Josephine when the worker showed me into a small room, the size of a closet, and handed me a wrap with snaps.

What am I supposed to do with this?

She read my thoughts saying "Hang your clothes on that hook, and put the wrap on," and then left.

Why?

I struggle with my pants, then lose all hope when my arm tangles in my shirt.

"Oh, you're not dressed yet?" The lady says when back. "What's taking so long? Here, let me help," and proceeds to undress the upper part of my body. I struggle, not wanting my clothes off. "Now, come on you have to get undressed," she keeps saying.

Why?

When dressed in the upper wrap she sets me down saying, "Now watch the video on breast cancer, and I'll be back to get you."

I sit with other women in the room watching a video on breast cancer. *Why? I don't have breast cancer. I have Alzheimer's. What does breast cancer have to do with Alzheimer's?*

Not liking where I am, I get up and walk toward the other room looking for Josephine and Sally. I'm stopped immediately by another woman, "No, you can't go out dressed like that," she says.

I back up into the room with women dressed like me, in wraps.

The first woman comes saying, "Okay Carol, we're ready for you now.

Ready for what?

She holds my hand, leading me to a machine that looks familiar, but one I haven't seen in a long time. She takes my arm out of the wrap and puts my breast on a slab. Without warning another piece of the machine comes down squashing my boob.

"Rata, Rata, Rata," I say, but she doesn't listen, like everyone doesn't listen. I repeat again, "Rata, rata, rata." *I'm in pain. It hurts.*

Nothing. She goes somewhere else while I'm stuck to the machine. I can't move, and start to cry. I never cry.

Finally she comes back, "Okay, we're done."

When unstuck, I ask, "Sha, sha, sha?" *Why are you checking my breasts and not checking my brain, to see if I've had a wrong diagnosis?* But she doesn't listen.

***

When Rose got the phone call saying Carol didn't have breast cancer, she blew a gasket. "Mammogram. Are you crazy? Why would you put her through that? Carol has Alzheimer's not Breast Cancer."

***

Carol is in the Alzheimer's locked down unit of a nursing home. She thinks Rose put her there to help others. She thinks Rose is ill, that's why they're not together. The holes she jumps over are black tiles, as she paces all day long up and down halls. Rose has gotten call after call saying Carol is hard to handle and needs private aides. Carol sleeps little, except for cat naps when she winds up in someone else's room, or an aide finds her and brings her back to her room. She eats little and is losing weight at a steady pace. It's five years now since the diagnosis. Rose cared for her four years, until Carol threw her through the shower doors. She then became afraid of her dear friend, the one who wouldn't hurt a flea, the one who talked to animals and plants, the one she loved. Rose herself is having a hard time without

Carol. Depression has taken over completely. She feels lost most of the time, the same way Carol feels lost in the nursing home. Carol at least wants to go somewhere, maybe the home she knew as a child, but Rose doesn't want to go anywhere. She doesn't want to live without Carol by her side.

But she tells the home, "Hire private aides," and writes an extra check each month for $4,000 out of Carol's trust account. At $10,000 a month for Carol's care, Rose is concerned how long the money will last.

Chapter 6

Sitting eating in the dining room, Carol sees aide, Darlene, talking with other aides. I bet she's coming my way to stick me on the commode for an hour.

Funny thing about this Alzheimer's, you still know what's going on even though those who care for you think you don't. They think you're out of your mind, or an infant. Well, fat chance. I'm no baby.

I chat with Millie, feeling sorry for her, because she can't do much sitting in a wheelchair. I like Millie, we have things in common, like understanding one another. But I still feel sorry for her. I notice the aides leave her just sitting in the hall, until they come and take care of her. Aides, Jennifer and Vivian, are nice to her, but they really don't understand what it's like to live here day and night. At least I can move about, but Millie is stuck where she's put.

"Sha, sha, sha," I say, *Here comes fatso-bug-shirt-aide,* and Millie smiles. I'm glad I gave her a smile.

I'm ready for her, Millie. She thinks I can't see her. How could you miss her? She's the size of three city blocks. And her butt? When she walks down the hall she could hold two barrels of water on each hip. Up and down they go, swishing and swashing from side to side with each step.

Millie laughs out loud, and I'm glad I made it happen.

"Have we eaten all our lunch, Ms. Carol?" asks fatso Darlene.

Who does she think she's talking to? *Ms. Carol ... ha.* She only says that when others are around, and they think she's showing respect for the patient. Which I know, she doesn't have.

Fatso takes my tray, then says, "Come Carol, time for potty."

Bye Millie.

She pulls my chair back then lifts under my arms and pulls me up. Facing me she pulls me down the hall.

"Good, Ms. Carol. We're going to go potty."

In my room she closes the door then retrieves a new pair of pants and an adult diaper from my dresser. I guess I dropped some sauce on my pants. *Didn't see that before.* She doesn't put the dirty pants in the laundry bag, instead places them in 'her' bag that she keeps in my closet. So she's the one stealing my clothes. Rose left me with lots of clothes from home.

I know, because I was a clothes-aholic. I loved clothes—expensive clothes. Most of them came from Palm Beach. Lilly's my favorite. I wear them here. But they seem to disappear after each wearing. I never thought about Darlene, but I see now she's the one stealing.

There she goes taking a nip from that bottle she keeps in her bag. Wonder what's in it? I've seen lots of pill bottles in her bag, almost as many as they give me to take at night.

After potty, and anything else she did, Fatso Darlene is gone and I finally get a chance to walk. Where's the exit? Oh, there it is, I see the sign down the end of the hall. I push the door—nothing. Still broken. Push again, harder. "Rata, Rata, Rata." *Let me out. I need to go.* I give up and look for another way out. I walk up the hall to the desk, where women in white uniforms are, with others who have bugs crawling all over their shirt, brown, red, blue. Why do they wear those shirts? Can't they see the bugs?

I walk past the desk, doors slide open, and I walk fast through them. What's that noise? Fire Engines coming. Crouched in the corner I hear the engine blaring. An aide takes my arm. "Rata, rata, rata." *leave me be*, I say.

"Come with me Carol, let's go this way."

She does something with the lit numbers on the wall where the doors were, and Fire Siren stops. I go with her to the desk. She gives me a cup of water, and puts something in my mouth. I spit it out. She retreats to the cart, then puts liquid in my mouth. It tastes good, sweet. I swallow. She leads me to the blue drape room. My eyes are heavy, they weren't before. I lay down. I'm so tired.

I fall asleep, but when my eyes open a woman is kneeling on a small rug in the middle of my room, facing the window.

I walked the halls all morning looking for a way out when a nurse decided I needed a relaxant. I took the liquid only because she waited for me to swallow.

Now, I watch *this* woman with a white scarf wrapped around her head and neck. Only her face shows. While kneeling, she bends over at the waist, her head and arms down to the floor while she chants something. *Praying?* Didn't she go to church this morning, like Rose and I used to?

This isn't church. It's a place you come to help people, but I'm tired of helping people, and all I hear is yelling and cursing from others.

Why is this woman kneeling and rambling on and on in my room?

Chapter 7

While Rose sat in the doctor's office waiting her turn, she overheard a woman talk about her ex-husband having dementia. Rose's ears perked up as the woman told another person sitting next to her.

"He's lost his short term memory. His heart stopped beating for fifteen minutes. No oxygen went to his brain. His brain swelled, but has come back to normal now. But, he doesn't remember his wife or the child they have. He only remembers me, his first wife, and our children."

Rose listened amazed. How does someone lose twenty-five years of their life? Just blot it out? What does his 'now' wife feel, and their child?

The woman went on telling this fascinating story:

"He said to our daughter, 'I want to see Pop Pop.'

"Dad, Pop Pop is dead. He died seventeen years ago."

'Oh no. Why didn't you tell me?' he asked.

Then he asked about his brother, who also had passed away and again he was mad no one had told him. The daughter said, "We did tell you." And he went on being mad, at something he didn't remember.

Rose sat, thinking, why did you tell him? You should have known it would upset him. But even his doctor said it was okay to tell him the truth.

The woman went on, "They put him in hyperbaric chamber, into a comma, so his brain would come back to normal size. They said there's no brain damage."

Rose wondered about that, No brain damage, but he can't remember the last twenty-five years of his life?

Rose wondered how much doctors knew about the brain, and didn't think very much, listening to this story.

Rose thought about Carol, wishing she had been diagnosed like this, instead of the doctor saying, "Dementia, of an Alzheimer's type."

The woman was called in to see another doctor in the same office and left Rose's presence.

Interesting, Rose thought.

When the male nurse led me down the hall to a room, I asked how he was. "Fine," he said, but running way behind schedule.

"Why's that?" I asked.

"Because, He," pointing to the doctor, "talks too much"

"Well, that's not a bad thing," I said.

"No, not for you guys," said the nurse.

"You mean he talks too much to his patients?" I asked.

"Yeah. We don't have the time. He spends too much time talking to patients," and wiped his nose with his arm.

My first thought: flu season, I sure hope he uses gloves when he checks my vitals.

"Talking to his patients is a good thing. Too bad he has to spend so much time on the computer. He *should* talk to his patients. He reminds me of my doctor growing up. He came in and asked, "how you doing?" and struck up a conversation. Otherwise how can a doctor know what's wrong with his patients, unless he talks to them?"

The nurse looked at me. After all there was a fifty year difference between us, so how could he understand the olden days? What a shame.

I was glad when the doctor came in and said, "How are you, Rose?"

I smiled and said, "Not too bad, Doc."

Chapter 8

Something new happened. Almost every day I have someone in my room. Two people, maybe. They don't do much. Most don't really talk. They read a lot and watch soap operas on my television. I'm not sure what their purpose is, but I'm sure they get paid for doing whatever it is they do.

When I walk the halls they don't go with me. They say they're tired and sleep in the recliner or pray on a rug. Most of the time they're not even around. Wish I could get a job like that.

***

There's the glass door. I liked being there last time. I push the door. It dosen't open. *I opened it last time*. I look through the glass and see: flowers, patio furniture, and the iron-gate I climbed over. *I'm sure I got out here.*

Finally I give up and stare ... nice blue flowers, pink hanging baskets. It's so pretty.

Aide, Vivian, takes my hand and leads me away. She brings me to the bird cage, pulling up a chair for me to sit.

"Sha sha, Sha," I say. *Thank you, Vivian.*

She points and describes the birds, "See Carol, that one is a finch, and the one over there is a sparrow."

I know that. Doesn't she know I was a bird watcher? I spent hours in nature watching birds. Mother and I would watch ducks and swans on the pond. In Florida, with Rose, I saw egrets, plovers, blue herons, white herons, Ibis, and many others. I was a *good* bird watcher. All the watercolor and oils in the house were different birds and ducks. Woodduck, my favorite, because it has so many different colors.

"Sha, sha, sha, sha, sha," *I was a bird watcher*, I tell Vivian.

Vivian nods and gives me a kiss on the cheek. She's nice, but I don't think she really understands … maybe a little.

She hurries off to help someone drinking out of the water fountain. Every time the woman goes to drink, it stops spurting. Vivian pushes the bar and water spurts out. The woman bends down and drinks. Why doesn't the woman know to do that? I do. Vivian's always helping someone.

Chapter 9

I hear on television something called Tau protein, not plaque, may cause Alzheimer's, but then I hear losing one's smell is a sign of Alzheimer's. I haven't lost my smell yet. I can smell the dirty diapers in the hall bin, then the deodorant spray to cover up the bad smell. They also say something in the eyes can show Alzheimer's. Again, I have great eye sight, and don't need glasses, but Rose does. They say an electrical brain implant can stop it. They have drugs, which do nothing. Some work a short time, but then the person is back to where they started or further down the Alzheimer's path. Some even say too much sugar can cause Alzheimer's. I like sweets, always have, especially chocalotta ice cream. They also say not enough exercise can cause Alzheimer's. Well, little do they know. I've exercised all my life: played golf, played tennis, swam, biked, walked, and still do. So much for that theory. They say doing puzzles can ward off Alzheimer's. Well, again, how many puzzles have I done? Hundreds, and I was diagnosed with Alzheimer's.

My feeling? There's something in the water, air, dirt, or growth of our food. Something we cannot control.

Others who speak my language, diagnosed with Alzheimer's, feel the same way. Something else is causing Alzheimer's, or we were diagnosed wrong.

***

There's always something going on, a function of some kind. This morning after watching television, we saw a children's concert, twenty-five at least, dressed in blue and white. The boys wore blue jackets with white pants and girls blue skirts and white shirts. It was the first time I had seen them, but my friends say they come often.

Now aide, Marissa, wakes me from my nap saying, "Better use the potty, we have to go downstairs."

Downstairs? Downstairs for what? "Rata, rata rata."

Marissa leads me to the bathroom, where I sit thinking. *Downstairs? Maybe we're going to see singing children again? It was wonderful this morning. Why can't we do that more often? Maybe we're doing it now. Goody.*

Marissa thinks my blouse needs changing, and here I thought I looked fine. No spots from drinking milk at lunch, or any other spots. But she does her changes and I can't wait to see the children, and hear the music.

She says something to the head nurse at the front desk, and then we get in the room with slide back doors. She does something to the side buttons and no siren sounds. *I need to learn those buttons.*

I feel the room drop, and then doors slide back. Marissa takes my hand, saying, "This way Carol." As I head right thinking we're going to see the singing children. I'm sure we went right this morning.

But maybe they're singing in a different place now, to the left.

We walk a way down the hall then stop at a half glass door. I look inside. Someone's seated at a desk, and other doors show inside the room. This doesn't look like the place with singing children.

Once inside the person at the desk says, "Carol. Right?" and Marissa answers, "Yes."

"Two-thirty appointment? asks desk-woman, "Right? Good, there's no wait." She then walks me into another room, where I see a funny looking chair, one I've seen before. A short man dressed in a white shirt jacket says, "Hello Carol." I nod. He offers his hand for me to sit in the chair, which I do. He helps with my legs, putting them up, so I'll be comfortable. He starts reclining the chair and suddenly bad memories come. I jump to a sitting position. "Rata, Rata, Rata?" *What's going on here? Where's the singing children?*

He and the woman push me down. "Rata, rata, rata." *Don't push me. I don't want to be here.*

Next to the chair I see shiny instruments, picks, pliers, tiny mirrors, and something else attached to a metal string. Then it hits. I remember—drill. I didn't like them when I was young, and I didn't like them with Rose.

I jump up. The man tries coaxing me down. I grab him around the neck. Easy, he's very short.

I get up, my arm around his neck. "Rata, rata rata." *Come, I'll take you to the singing children down the hall.* Marissa and the lady say something I can't quite make out and the man mumbles into my side.

Remember, I'm fast. They have a hard time keeping up, but soon others are trying to unclasp my arm.

"She went to the dentist and then dragged him all the way to the auditorium," I hear Marissa say when we are upstairs. The aides and nurses laugh. So I guess something funny happened.

Chapter 10

I'm downstairs at the ice cream parlor with Rose. *Yes*, she finally came. She must have been really sick. She says something about not visiting me so I could get used to who's taking care of me. I don't need anyone to take care of me. I can take care of myself.

Rose orders chocalotta ice cream. *Yippie*, my favorite, I haven't had it in ages. We go outside to the pond. I like that. Ducks and Geese hang around the water. If you watch closely you can see fish jump out of the water, sunning their bellies, then dive back in. Funny they know to do that. I guess nature takes care of itself better than humans care for themselves. Or maybe God takes care of them.

We sit on the bench under the overhanging tree. The tree keeps the sun out of my eyes. I once was a sun worshiper, but not now. I hardly ever see the sun, except when aides, Jennifer or Vivian, take me outside, which doesn't happen often. But I'm happy to have them.

Rose hands me a cup of ice cream, but I can't hold the spoon. It's too small and keeps falling out of my hand. Rose helps, spooning ice cream into my mouth. I can't open my mouth fast enough. I love ice cream, chocalotta especially.

Rose asks, "Are you happy, Carol?"

How do I answer that? *No. I'm not happy. I want to go home,* I say in my words. I tell her about the abuse that goes on here. But Rose doesn't understand.

"Ooh, did you see the fish jump out of the water?" she asks.

Well, of course I did. And I saw the two before that one. *Do you see the turtle on the bank sunning himself?* I say. But she doesn't answer, which tells me she doesn't understand what I've asked.

Done eating I throw the cup under the bench.

"No, Carol," Rose says, and reaches for the cup, throwing it in a big can across from us.

I guess I was supposed to throw it in there, and not under the bench. Next time I'll remember.

She tells me an old friend, Edith, says hello. I don't have a friend named Edith. Maybe it's her friend? She says our neighbors say hello. I remember them. Ruth is a doll. She bakes cakes and cookies and brings them to us for us to try. *I want to go back home and have Ruth's cookies.* But Rose doesn't understand.

"Let's take a walk around the pond," Rose says.

I'm up in a flash, hearing the word 'walk'. I love walking, always have. But Rose walks too slow for me. I'm ahead of her, even though she has my hand. I want to walk fast. I want to walk home.

"Slow down, Ca. You're going too fast for me."

But I can't. Everything tells me fast: golf, swimming, walking, biking. Fast. That's me.

Uh oh, she's pulling me toward the back door. *I don't want to go in there. I like it outside.* "Rata," *No.*

"Carol, we need to go upstairs."

"Rata, Rata, Rata, Rata," I say. *I can't go back. I don't want to. The people in there are bad.* Jennifer and Vivian are the only nice ones. A few others, but the bug-shirt women are bad. They don't let me finish meals. They push and pull me, hurt my arms. They leave bruises on me. You should have seen the black and blue I got from Fatso. It was bigger than a baseball.

"C'mon Carol," Rose says. And I go, not to upset her. I have a feeling Rose is sick and needs to leave.

Okay, I'll go, this time.

Upstairs she kisses me goodbye and leaves through the little room with sliding doors and siren sounds. But no siren sounds when Rose gets in.

Chapter 11

Walking down the hall Carol sees Millie. "Hi, Millie. How you doing?"

Millie answers in our language, "I'm fine, how about you?"

"Oh, I'm good. I just want out of this place. I've tried two Exits and both doors are broken."

Millie says there's another door, "It has a latch on it that's hard to turn. If you turn the latch, and push at the same time, the door will open. But don't let anyone see you."

I go where Millie tells me and turn the latch. The door opens. I mouth my 'thank you' to Millie.

It is a different door, one you'd never know is a door. But I find my way downstairs to sunlight, driveway, garbage cans and trucks parked.

I see a wooded area and head that way.

This is nice, trees, bushes, and air to breathe, different from that upstairs dungeon.

Happy to be out, Carol walks fast and falls into sticker bushes, getting scrapes on her arms and face. She hears frogs and ducks, and heads toward the sound.

Almost to the pond two men dressed in white overalls grab her.

"Rata, Rata, Rata," Carol yells, *Leave me alone.*

"Come with us, Carol. You shouldn't be out here."

"Rata, Rata, Rata" *Yes I Can.*

But they're stronger and larger and soon she's back in her room, bandaged up with liquid in her mouth. She has no choice but to swallow. In minutes she's asleep.

Little did Carol know the camera outside picked up her image.

***

"Where did you get those bruises?" Rose asks.

Carol tries answering but can't, she's too out of it to even walk.

Rose goes to the front desk. "Why is she so drugged and full of scrapes?"

She learns Carol got out and fell in bushes, "That's why she has scrapes," the aide says. "We had to sedate her. She kept fighting us."

"You had to sedate her? What kind of home is this if you can't keep an eye on your patients? Maybe she was better off home, instead of here." And Rose walks away mad.

Chapter 12

As I pass Sophie's room I hear her moaning. The door is closed part way, only a slit-light shines through. I ease it open more, and see two teenage-aide-helpers have hoisted Sophie's naked body in the air. A closer look tells me the redhead is putting something in Sophie's poop hole. The other dark girl jiggles Sophie's breasts. Sophie moans louder.

I yell, "Rata Rata. Rata Rata." *Stop that. Stop that.*

Turning, seeing me, the redhead says, "Oh don't worry about her, she's nuts. She doesn't know what's going on. She can't even talk, so she can't tell anyone. Get. Out." she yells to me.

I back out the door but first see Sophie look my way. *Tell someone*, her eyes relay.

In the hall I look both ways, no one there. I have to tell someone, like Sophie said. Good thing we can talk with our eyes. I head to the front desk. Nurse in white. I'll tell her.

"What's up Carol? Why are you so upset?"

Twice I repeat, "Rata, Rata, Rata, Rata." *Sophie's in trouble*. But she takes my hand. *No, they're abusing Sophie*. She leads me to the piano room. "Rata, Rata, Rata," I yell. *Sophie needs help*. But the nurse doesn't believe or understand.

Brain is in the hall and I tell him. He understands, but doesn't believe me. *I'm not kidding Brain. I saw it. Those teenage-aides that come to help out were abusing Sophie*.

"Well, we have to get rid of them. Right?"

I look at him, "Sha."*Right*.

Back in the television room: Millie, Marti, John, Stanley and Josephine are sitting. I tell them what I saw in Sophie's room. They had a feeling this was happening but haven't said anything, afraid of getting in trouble.

Well, we have to do something about this. It's wrong.

They agree. Stanley says, "But what can *we* do? No one understands us or will believe us."

I'll think of something, Carol says, in language they understand.

Chapter 13

"Okay Carol, it's poop time," Darlene says, while trying to yank me off the bed. The PA system blares, "Darlene, come to the desk."

"Oh shit. What the hell do they want?" she says. "Be right back, Dumbo," and leaves.

No way is Fatso Darlene going to get away with how she treats me. I'll make her pay. I'm tired of Fatso slamming a cold wet cloth into my face, saying she's washing me. I'm tired of Ms. Hispaniola wiping my behind, digging into sores she's made. I'm tired of Blondie shoving pureed chicken in my mouth making me choke. I'm tired. Period. It's time to fight back, and fight back now, the only way I know.

I'll take care of myself. I don't need Rose to take care of me. I could take care of her, if she'd let me.

While Fatso's out of the room, Carol slides her hand along the back of the bed, until she reaches the hidden pouch she made, full of pills. When nurses gave her pills she stored them in her cheek, then spit them in her hand, holding them for her little pouch. Now she goes to the closet and finds the bottle Fatso drinks from, and puts a handful of pills in it. She shakes the bottle a little. *Good.* One more shake for good luck.

Carol's sitting on the bed when Fatso comes in saying, "Those shitheads don't know what they're doing. I can't wait to get out of this ass-hole place."

Oh, pretty soon, Carol thinks.

Fatso pulls my arms to stand, but I don't budge. She tries again. I stay seated. I'm still strong. After all, Rose told me how strong I was when she fed me all those great meals, trying to cure me of this disease, which I probably don't even have.

She pulls my arms again. Nope. Nowhere.

Finally, disgusted she says, "Okay, stay there idiot," and goes to the closet.

I watch her take the bottle out of her bag. She opens it and drinks.

Good, drink more.

She usually takes a sip or two and puts it back, but this time she drinks a long time. She must be really mad.

Fatso wipes her mouth on the back of her hand, closes the closet doors, then heads toward me.

She pulls my arms up. Then pulls again, but this time not as forcefully. She puts her hands on her hips, then with one hand, wipes the sweat on her forehead. She sits on the bed shaking her head. Deciding she needs a drink of water, she reaches for the pitcher on my night stand and looks at me. I smile. "Whaa yu do?" she slurs, and drops the pitcher.

Getting up, she weaves then falls on her knees, like the praying woman with head and neck scarf, but different.

Oops, bye bye fatso.

On bended knee she tries getting up, then falls flat. I watch her back move up and down in time with her breathing.

I wait. I wait more.

Finally, no movement. No breath.

One down.

I have to get out of here. If they find out I got rid of her, they'll send me to jail, and lord knows I don't want to go to jail. That could be worse than here. If that's possible.

Good, no camera in my room. After seeing my bruises that day Rose thought about hiding a camera on the dresser under the lamp, good thing she didn't.

I leave Fatso on the floor and head for the television room. My friends are there, drinking juice.

"Hi, Marti, Sally, John, Josephine. How is everyone?"

"You're looking mighty chipper. What's up?" John says.

"Oh nothing. Just wondered what you all were doing."

We chat about the news on television, how bad it is. "Nothing happy nowadays, like the olden days. I want to go back to radio days, Amos and

Andy and Jack Benny show. Now it's war, hunger, killings, and terror attacks," Marti says.

"Not to mention what goes on here. I don't know what the aides get paid, but some are very mean. The one I had last night, smacked me because I wouldn't turn over," Sally adds. "The Hispanic one, I forget her name. She gave me a shower and I thought she used a horse brush on me."

"You mean Marissa," John answers. "You should have slapped *her*, Sally. You're good at that."

I listen wanting to tell them they won't have to worry about Fatso anymore. I took care of her, but I don't let on. Not yet.

Later I told Millie, only because I knew she wouldn't tell anyone, and I was bursting to tell someone and she's my good friend, a connected friend, kind of like what I had with Rose. *Where is she anyway?* I hope not very sick, she hardly comes to see me.

Brian wheels over and asks, "So who's next on your list, the teenage helpers?"

"Sha?" I ask. "Rata, rata, rata?" *What are you talking about?*

"You know perfectly well what I'm speaking of. Your rusty bucket list for those you don't like."

I get up, "Rata, Rata." *Goodbye Brian*, wondering how he knows.

I'm sure Millie didn't tell. How does Brian know? Has he been snooping around my room, behind my bed?

Not far down the hall who do I see? None other than next one on my rusty bucket list, as Brain calls it.

"Come Carol, time for changing and a nap," Marissa says.

But when we get to my room the door is closed. Marissa opens the door and peeks in. "Close The Door," someone yells. "Take Carol somewhere else."

I guess they found Fatso.

Keeping a close watch on my hall, a short time later I see people outside the door. Something's on a table, more likely some body, and they're wheeling it down the end of the hall and disappear.

I'm glad Fatso's gone. Even others are happy she's gone when they find out. Brian thanked me over and over for getting rid of her. I'm not sure how he knows I'm the one who got rid of her. I'll have to keep my eyes and ears open. News travels fast.

Chapter 14

Today's breakfast consisted of oatmeal, toast, orange juice, and coffee. It would have been nice if I'd had a chance to eat it. But again they wanted us out of the dining room early. Why? I have no idea.

I want out of this place.

No use going to the Exit sign that way, the door doesn't open, and the other door has cameras outside. I remember that one. I'll try the other hall. Half way down the hall sits Millie, as always, waiting for some aide to come to her needs.

"Sha, Sha" *Hi Millie.*

Hi Carol. Where you headed?

Nowhere really. Just looking for a way out of this place.

You might want to try the door at the end of this hall, Millie says.

I look down the hall. "Sha, sha, sha" *I've been there. The door's always locked.*

If you go just past the Exit sign down to the window at the end of the hall, next to it you'll see another door. It goes to the kitchen.

Oh, okay. Thanks Millie.

I walk almost to the window and see a door I didn't know was there. It is different. Flush to the wall, not like others, no small window on it, and no exit sign above. I push. Nothing. I push again. Nothing. Then notice a hook and eye latch. I unhook and pull. It opens. Odd, none of the doors open into the hall. They all push out into stairwells. I look down the hall, Millie smiles. I nod, thank you.

In front of me is a stairwell, but something different. A small escalator.

When I step on the elevated stairs they move downward. I'm going somewhere, but who knows where? I hold the rail, afraid of falling down moving stairs. I pass another door, and another. I'll get off the next door, but it stops at the end. I get off in a large room, basement maybe.

Canvas bins everywhere. Ten at least. I inch closer to a bin and look inside. Clothes. Lots of clothes. *My Lilly. How did it get here? I haven't seen it in weeks.* I pull it out of the bin and tuck it under my arm.

I see boxes of food, old, smelly food. What are they going to do with this?

Walking close to the wall, I see light showing under it. This must be a way out. Is it a push or pull door? I try pulling, it doesn't budge. Try pushing. Wha-la. I push again, further.

I hear people talking and crouch down. Where am I? I see light, but not outside light.

I listen. What are they saying? Something about so and so having to leave, and take their things with them. Somebody I don't know. The name is not familiar. Renee or Rinee, something like that, must be a worker.

I open the door more. Where are they? I hear them but can't see them.

I inch further.

At the wall, voices come from above me. From a large screened fluorescent light. A very bright light.

Looking around I see stretchers with sheets over them. I walk to the nearest one and lift the sheet.

Oh my god, someone's dead.

It looks like the woman on my floor. But I'm not sure. Her skin's grey. I guess this is what dead white people look like. Lips purple ... kind of purple-blue. I saw her at breakfast and thought she looked fine, chatting with her table mates. How'd she die so fast?

I lift the sheet next to her, *Yikes, Fatso.* Now she doesn't look bad, but why isn't she with her loved ones in a funeral home? She's lost a lot of weight I see. Maybe they sucked fluid out of her or gave her a tummy tuck ... *ha, ha* ... I like that.

Uh oh, someone's yelling, "Why'd you put her in there stupid?"

"Because that's the only free space. There wasn't any other place. We're all filled up," says another man.

"Well, get her the hell out of there, and put her in the furnace."

Furnace? and look behind me. Big massive heater, one we had in olden days for coal and wood, but this one's taller and wider.

"Get going. Do it now, before they find her."

I see part of the wall move, slide back, almost like the room upstairs, doors slide into walls and sirens blare. No sirens now.

I have to get out of here before they see me. I run to the moving stairs I took down, not looking back. Riding the stairs, I make it to floor number three. My floor. Millie's still sitting in the hall.

"You're not going to believe what I saw, Millie." She questions with her eyes. But I can't say, because here comes Jennifer.

"Well, hi Carol. How are you? What's that under your arm?" Jennifer asks.

"Sha, sha, sha," I say. *It's my Lilly shirt.* And she nods and smiles. Doesn't she understand? *I found the lady I saw at breakfast, and Fatso, my clothes, and food.*

"Nice chatting with you Carol. Let's get you changed Millie." And they head toward Millie's room.

I hang my Lilly shirt in the blue-draped room. The one Rose likes so much. I'm tired. I'll lie here and think about what I saw, and what to do next. Number one: *Don't tell Brain.*

***

Marti found a way out. Literally walked away from this place. Only problem, they found him miles away walking alongside the road. *He* knew where he was going, no one else did. I'll have a talk with Marti, see how he got out, or was it the same way I got out when cameras picked me up.

Chapter 15

They used to say Alzheimer's hits old people, but now young people are getting Alzheimer's dementia, Lewy Body dementia, Frontal Lobe dementia and other dementias. I even heard on the news a young girl has Picks disease—dementia. Even diabetes and heart disease can cause dementia. I wonder how many dementias there are, and how many people are wrongly diagnosed?

On television I saw a 72 year old woman went missing. They found her, but she died two days later in the hospital. I guess they didn't find her soon enough.

When I get out next time, they won't find me. I need to make a plan, and follow it. I wonder were all these lost people looking for Home?

***

I remember when my blood pressure was up and my heart beats were off. Rose took me to the emergency room. I was hooked up to a monitor and my blood pressure read 190/101 and pulse 90. I watched the monitor read my heart beats, and they just didn't look right to me or Rose. She asked the ER nurse, "Why is the bottom line dipping so low and not coming back on time like others." "Oh, she's throwing PVC's," the nurse said. "No problem. It happens sometime."

I laid there, them poking and prodding my belly and anything else they could poke. Then I was taken for a CTscan of the brain, making sure I had no brain bleeds. Then they did a chest x-ray, looking for blood clots in the lungs and an EKG.

After two hours they took blood. That hurt the most. One of the ER nurses apparently hadn't passed taking blood course in school, because she tried three times jamming needles into both arms, unable to get blood. Finally Rose said, "Would you please find someone else." And she did, someone who went from room to room only drawing blood. That was her job, draw blood. She came, introduced herself, and asked my name. I told her, "Sha." and she looked at Rose. "Carol," Rose said. And the women understood. She didn't understand me.

For four hours I laid on an uncomfortable ER bed, freezing to death while Rose asked for more blankets.

They gave me a blood pressure pill, saying, "See your doctor in the next three to five days."

We both came home tired. We had lunch falling asleep watching television.

I wonder why I don't have high blood pressure attacks here. Or maybe I do, and nobody cares to check. Maybe that's not important anymore.

Interesting why I remember old days and forget the new days.

***

I run in to Stanly in the hall and relay the news I heard, "Stanley, did you hear Sally's husband shot her, and then shot himself? They found a note next to his body, saying he couldn't live without her anymore."

"Not only that, Carol. Someone went for a walk yesterday, and didn't come back."

"Really? You want to go for a walk?"

"Sure," he says. "Whenever you're ready."

"Great, I'll let you know. I'm sick of what goes on here. No one listens. They just do what *they* want. You'd think if they wanted to learn about Alzheimer's/Dementia, they'd ask us, and not read some old book. I don't understand why the staff is so unfriendly, except for a few. Why do they handle us like objects, instead of real people?"

"I don't know, Carol. I'm sick of it also. You'd think they'd be kind, knowing we have a problem, but no, they just do they're thing. Whatever that is. Mostly they're texting on their phones. How the establishment allows that is beyond me. If I would have done that when I worked I'd have gotten fired. But then again they didn't have texting when I worked."

An aide stops our chatting, taking Stanley for his shower. "See ya, Carol."

I yell, "Rata, Rata, Rata." *Good luck, Stanley. Don't let her give you sleeping pills.*

I walk away headed in the direction Millie last told me, passed the Exit sign. *Wonder how the runaway got out?*

I'll miss Sally. I liked her. She was tough and knew what was going on. She probably tried telling her husband, but he didn't understand. Or he couldn't take seeing his wife with Alzheimer's anymore. Too bad he didn't understand her.

Aide Marissa saw me talking to Stanley, then gave me the pills I told him not to take. I moved them with my tongue to my cheek, sipped water, and swallowed. Everyone I see who takes pills, winds up slumped over in chairs or in bed. Marissa thought I took them. Little does she know, I spit them in my hand and held them for my pouch. *These may be yours, Marissa.*

Chapter 16

I'm down the elevated stairs. I'm not afraid this time. I push/pull the door that has the light under, only to find the room stripped bare. No bins. No clothing. No food.

Now, where's that sliding door? I tap walls until I see a slit of light. That's it. I tap more, near the bottom. The wall slides back.

I'm not lifting sheets this time looking for bodies. They'll be in the furnace soon. I'm sure.

No voices. They must be taking a lunch break. Good thing I ate early.

Looking in a corner, I see double doors. The push out kind. I push one side. It opens. Day-light. Real, day-light. It must be the back of the facility. I make my way into the woods, thinking, this must be where they found James. It had spread through the facility like wild fire. James walked out and wasn't found for months. They found his clothes, sitting next to a tree, along with his bones, as if he'd been just sitting there. No one had bothered to look in that spot. I wonder did they even look. His body was gone, eaten by animals we suspected. They collected his bones and lay them on a stretcher. It's unbelievable the things that go on, that the outside world doesn't know, or wouldn't want to know.

I'll make sure I don't get found like James.

Away from the building, I'm out. Now what? Which way? Right, left, forward, definitely not back. I know what's there. People drug you and hurt you.

I turn right, then left, nothing. In front of me is a dirt path. I follow it.

I walk, trees hang low and birds chirp. I'm on the right path, I know. Something inside me says: this is the path to freedom.

I need to get as far away from that place as possible. They must *not* find me.

But how will Rose find me when she visits? Well, she'll have to understand, I had to get away. I only hope she's not ill, and if so, that she'll get better.

After walking a while, I decide to sit on the side of the path. Frogs are close. I hear them. They must be near water, I'm very thirsty. I follow their voice.

Vines, sticker bushes scrape my arms as I follow frog voices. A pond appears in the open. I kneel at the edge, cup my hands and drink. Not great tasting, but drink until I can't drink anymore. Herons, Ibis, Egrets, green Herons, crowd the water's bank. I watch, bringing memories of Rose and I on golf courses, egrets sat on over hanging limbs and herons searched for fish at pond's edge.

What went wrong? Why did we stop playing golf?

I get up and get back to walking, this time not looking for an Exit sign. This time, my path forward.

Car horns. This must be the way. Closer, closer. Then literally one step out of the woods, I see lanes and lanes of cars. Some going one direction, others the opposite direction. A highway. No traffic lights. I stand a while figuring, what now? There is no forward. There's only left or right. Which way?

The afternoon sun is over the road, so that's gotta be south. I don't want to go that way. I'll go right. Walk along the highway. Why not? I used to see people do it all the time, walk the highway with their finger in the air. I'll try.

Walking, maybe half-an-hour, my finger in the air, a car finally stops. A woman shouts, "Get in."

I don't know her, but I get in. I can't stay out in the dark. Or can I?

"Hello dear," the woman says.

I nod my head, and say "Sha, Sha." She doesn't respond.

"Where you going to?" the woman asks.

"Sha, sha, sha," *home*, I answer.

The woman's quiet, then says, "So you're going to Savannah?"

Savannah? No. I don't want to go there. I was there a long time ago.

"Rata, Rata, Rata," I say, *I'm going home.*

"Well, I'm not going as far as Raleigh, but I'll take you to St. Augustine. That's my last stop," she says.

I guess that's not bad, and nod.

She turns on the radio, nice easy listening music, music that doesn't make my head spin, as the aides listen to in my room. Soon I'm sleeping, out of this world, and on my way home.

Chapter 17

At St. Augustine rest stop, Carol is dropped off by the nice woman. "Sha, sha, sha." *Nice meeting you,* Carol says, as the woman drives off.

Now what? Bathroom first, four hours is a long time without going. She looks and looks for a bathroom, but finds none, and winds up in the woods with her pants down. After business, she scrapes leaves and dirt over it, and walks away.

She sees a woman pushing a four wheel grocery cart coming from the same woods.

"Sha, sha, sha." *Hi, I'm Carol.*

The dark haired woman answers, "Hi I'm Verna. Nice to meet you Carol."

Carol sees Verna has lots of eye makeup on, mostly black, with some blue sparkles around her eyes, and heavy red lipstick and red blush cheeks. She's dressed nicely in a coat and scarf. In Verna's cart Carol notices blankets, pillow, sweaters, and can't figure why the coat? This is Florida, it doesn't get that cold, even though Carol has her favorite sweat suit on. Verna's talking and Carol understands her and Verna understands Carol, which makes them special. They understand each other, like her nursing home friends.

Carol decides to ask, "Verna, why do you wear such heavy makeup?"

"Oh, that. To tell you the truth most people don't talk to me because of it. They think I'm crazy wearing a lot of makeup. Men think I'm a hooker, and I throw them off making believe I can't speak English. You know, the kind of language you speak Carol."

"That's funny. I never thought of that." So people think I'm crazy because I don't speak english, English. Like Rose and workers at the nursing ... *better not tell that.*

"Where you headed Carol? I'm off to the bathroom to wash up," Verna says.

"Where's the bathroom? I must have missed it."

"Come, I'll show you. I use it every day, sometimes many times a day."

Carol and Verna walk a short distant to the building Carol was in before. This time Verna shows her the bathroom, sinks and even showers. *I won't need that.* Carol thinks. *But maybe now I might.*

"So where you going, Carol? You can wash the scrapes on your arms in the sink over there."

"Thank you Verna. Don't know yet where I'm going, maybe home, but maybe not, depends on where my path takes me."

Verna laughs, "Sounds like me. Follow your path ... I guess we have something in common."

Carol can't find the soap, and Verna helps by pushing the dispenser to soap Carol's hands.

"I'm going to take a shower, Carol. You can sit and wait over there, on the bench, if you like."

"I'm not going to shower. I did already early this morning, before I got on the road."

"You have a car?" Verna asks.

"No. My friend dropped me off. She's visiting friends then coming back to get me." *Had to think of something, besides walking away from a nursing home.*

After showering, Verna says, "Well, it's getting late. If your friend doesn't come, you can stay with me and the others. We'll walk back together."

I'd like that. I really don't want to be out in the dark, and no friend is coming back.

"Thank you Verna."

Chapter 18

Verna leads the way to a camp ground, deep into the woods.

Carol has never known homeless people, although she gave to charities helping the homeless, but now a dog circles her legs.

"This is Daisy, Carol. Our mascot."

Daisy sniffs my feet. I put my hand down for her to smell, letting her know I'm not an enemy, or anyone who'd hurt her. She sniffs and sniffs, then jumps up and down as if on a pogo stick. I pick her up and she gives kisses with her tongue. I've always loved dogs, all kinds, maybe not big, big dogs.

"Folks, I want you to meet Carol," Verna yells.

"Well, if Daisy welcomes you Carol, we do too," says a man dressed in overalls and a blue denim shirt. His hair is long, with a gray tinged beard. His eyes, the bluest I've ever seen.

"Thanks Frank, for the welcome," Verna says. "I'm sure it means a lot to Carol. She's been on the road a while. Her friend dropped her off and never came back, so maybe she can join us."

In minutes, others come patting me on the back and offering a hello hand. Nothing like nursing home welcomes, offering pills.

By eight o'clock I'd had two hot dogs and soda. Full to the brim, and now they roasted marshmallows in the fire, passing them around to all. Boy, this thing 'homeless' is not bad at all.

Lots of people to talk to, some speaking my language, and some not. I don't quite understand that.

Someone plays an old beat-up piano that someone else threw out, and Frank asks, "Howabout a dance Carol?"

I look at Verna. "Go ahead Carol. He doesn't ask everyone."

I got up from my sitting position, and soon Frank led me in a polka, while others joined in, singing the beer barrel polka. Why couldn't the nursing home be like this?

After the dance Frank asked if I wanted a smoke. I used to smoke, but stopped, don't remember why or when, but it sounded good and I hadn't lost my taste for it.

He took paper out of his pants pocket, put tobacco in, rolled it up, then licked the edge sealing it.

I took one inhale and blew it out. "No, Carol. Inhale and hold it, like this." And he held his breath.

"Okay." And tried his way.

Whoa, this wasn't any cigarette I'd smoked before. My head started buzzing and I felt light as a feather, flying like I could reach the clouds, if there were clouds. Being night I couldn't see a cloud in the sky. But the stars shined bright, and I was sure I could touch them if I tried.

Frank told me he came from a small town in Virginia. We had something in common. I had gone to college in Virginia, an all-girls school. He knew it well. "Good school," he said. "What'd you do afterward?"

I thought a moment, and everything came flooding back with each joint (as Frank called them) I smoked. I remembered my past life now better than ever before. I went to college and worked in the big city. Later I worked with Mom and Dad, then ran the business after Dad died and Mom had a stroke. I remembered it all: Semi Pro Golfer, especially Mom standing behind a tree taking pictures of me swinging a golf club. Daisy came and sat by my side, listening. I rubbed behind her ear and she tilted her head wanting more.

By ten o'clock Verna said she was tired and I was welcome to sleep in her tent. I took her up on the offer.

Not having any clothes made it hard, because the night was chilly. Verna offered a sweater and blanket. I thanked her, finding myself comfortable inside her tent on her blanket. And Daisy snuggled into my left side.

We talked a bit about the fun filled day I'd had and I soon drifted into never never land without a pill from an aide or nurse.

Rose came to mind and I wondered if they'd told her I was gone? Was she out looking for me?

This might be home for now, twenty-five tents deep in the woods, serving children, women and men.

Chapter 19

Rose wakes feeling the need to visit Carol, whether she wants to or not. She's trying to get along without Carol, have a life of her own, enjoy *something*. Alzheimer's has been tied around her neck for too long. She doesn't want to abandon Carol, but knows she needs time for herself, otherwise she will die before Carol. After one of her visits to the doctor, he said, "You can't care for Carol anymore. You're going to have a heart attack if you keep caregiving."

Rose listened and put Carol in a nursing home, but this day she feels the need to see her. She drives listening to music, knowing what lay ahead, the craziness of the disease.

Off the elevator she makes a right to the end of the hall, to the blue room, thinking Carol liked it so much, her favorite color. But Carol's not there and not walking the halls.

She stops an aide in the hall, "Where is Carol," and is surprised by the answer she gets. "What do you mean you can't find her?" Rose asks.

"I left her sleeping in her room, and when the next shift came on Carol was gone."

"Where the heck is she? How can you lose someone?"

The aide takes Rose to her superior where she asks the same question, "How the heck can you lose someone in a facility? You have cameras. Have you checked them?"

The superior makes a phone call finding news on Carol. Carol had gone out an old door never used, that doesn't have cameras.

Rose is livid. "How the hell can you lose someone in a locked down unit?" and goes off steamed. "I'll look for her myself," She yells over her shoulder. "Don't expect to get paid this month. In fact you might want to check tomorrow morning's headlines."

Chapter 20

Meanwhile Carol is having a great time at the homeless camp. People love her and treat her with kindness, not like the nursing home, where they yell, treat her unkindly and give pills.

One woman, Ester, is seventy years old and Carol wonders how she can be homeless? Why isn't her family caring for her? Why isn't government taking care of her with Social Security?

"Well, you see Carol it's like this. I have no family, and my social security check comes to $600 a month. That buys food, some clothing, and pays doctor bills. I have high blood pressure and take pills, so that's more money spent. I put some on a credit card, which grows every month. That takes up most of my check."

"How can that be, in this country?" Carol asks.

"I guess this country is not as good as it used to be," Ester says. "Plus everything you buy is too high. Food has gotten way overpriced. Milk alone cost three dollars a gallon. Toilet paper, that's really high, four dollars for four rolls of paper. I don't know how the companies get away with it, let alone live with themselves. It's a rich man's country. We used to grow vegetables and live off them in winter. Not anymore. Everything is for the young person, not the elderly. Soon they'll have free college, and the elderly won't have a roof or food. Like me. See that garden over there, at least we have fresh vegetables. Thank God for the folks here, otherwise I couldn't live."

Carol is in awe that someone this age should be homeless, living in a camp, and not have her own place. What's happened to this country? Is it only for the rich? Which I once was, she thinks. Maybe not rich, rich, but I could afford to play golf, belong to country clubs, go to lunch and dinners a few times a week. Maybe I was rich and didn't know it. I was well off, that I know. How can I afford the nursing home if I don't have money? Rose takes care of all that. My money will run out some day. I guess there's no security in this country. In fact, Rose is paying for my room now, and I'm not there. Boy, I bet she's mad.

"Ester, I hope things change for you and you can have your own little place, with a door knocker."

Ester laughs, "I doubt it Carol. But we can hope, can't we?"

Thank God for Verna and her tent, otherwise I'd be sleeping on the streets.

Weeks go by, Carol having happy times, Daisy jumping up wanting petting, and homeless friends offering her anything they have. No pureed foods, mashed together, like in the nursing home. She misses her clothes, but makes do with what is offered her.

Carol noticed the homeless were different colors and different religions. Why did everyone blend together here as One, when in the unhomeless world everyone fought each other? She'd heard on the news, all the time, at the nursing home, Whites were fighting Blacks and Spanish, Christians were fighting Jews and Muslims.

Here at homeless camp was the ideal way to live, everyone got along, sharing what little they had, with each other. This was a 'united' world.

Maybe the United Nations should learn by living in a Homeless camp. Maybe the United Nations should be in different countries, and not centered in the U.S.

Most children walked to school except for young ones, first and second graders. Mothers gave last address they lived, or chose an apartment building close to the school, saying they lived there.

One late afternoon we gathered around a handsome young boy named, Sam. He was going to his first junior prom and all had chipped in finding a dark blue suit, shirt, tie, socks and black wing tips. He could pass for a movie star, especially when

Donna gave him a haircut, and rubbed gel on his dark brown wavy hair.

He shined, inside an out, after sneaking into the large, store's employee bathroom, up the road, for a shower.

His mother had a hard time letting him go. She kissed him, saying, "Now, don't you come home too late. You hear?"

"Oh, Helen, let the boy go," Frank said. "He's a man now. Go on Sam, have a great time, and stay out as long as you want. I'll keep your mother busy dancing tonight."

We laughed, knowing how much Helen hated seeing her boy grow into a man. Others with middle school children knew their time was coming soon.

Frank *kept* Helen dancing that night, and then most of us went to sleep.

I don't know what time Sam came home, it was past my bed time. Verna and I talked, while Daisy cuddled against my side.

"They sure grow up fast, don't they Carol?"

I hadn't had any children and could only imagine what Helen was going through.

"Yes, they do," I answered sleepily, while rubbing Daisy behind the ear.

***

Early one morning, after weeks smiling, Carol hears truck noises. She peeks out of the tent and beckons Verna to come see. Truck plows, like snow plows, but there's no snow. It's Florida. The first five tents have been plowed under and friends are yelling, "NO. This is our home," and children stand crying. "No, don't do that. We live here."

"Get all you can hold, Carol, and let's get out of here."

Verna has her cart full, but Carol has only shopping bags, filled with sweaters, and some food and drinks, that she can carry.

"Hurry Carol. We need to get out of here, otherwise we're going to be plowed under too."

Carol runs with Verna and others, watching their homes get demolished. A news reporter is asking questions and Frank is answering. "We lived here. This was our home. How can they just come along and plow it under? What are we supposed to do now? You think the city is going to find us places to stay? I doubt it. They didn't before. It all costs money, and they don't want to spend any on us because we can't give anything back. After all how much tax can they collect from us?"

Chapter 21

Headlines: "Homeless Camp Demolished" with Frank, Verna and Carol's photo on TV. Seen at the nursing home, soon Carol is back in the blue room.

She's mad. She doesn't want to be there. She liked living at the homeless camp. She liked her friends, especially Daisy jumping up and down waiting to be petted. Daisy even slept with Carol when she wasn't standing guard against intruders. She tells her friends at the nursing home how some of the homeless understood her. *They spoke our language*. But she hears some have died at the nursing home while she was gone. She hears how the aides have been treating them.

"It hasn't changed, Carol. The aides have gotten worse. I heard from a few that they're not making any money and they'd rather work in burger places." Brain says. "Oh, and John is very ill. I think he's dying."

The worse news of all. "John dying". One of her first friends. What's happened since she left?

***

Rose visits, welcoming her back, letting Carol know she's still there for her. Carol tells Rose how bad it is living at the nursing home and how some of the homeless understood her, but Rose doesn't understand.

Chapter 22

I didn't know if aide Blondie was on tonight or not. I had seen her earlier mouthing off to one of my friends, thinking, *it's time, Blondie.*

We were in the television room watching news, as usual, when something came on of interest.

"Someone murdered in nursing home, bashed in head."

Um, could I bash in Blondie's head? No, too messy. That would be another Marissa. The teenagers were happy to see that, I'm sure. Although, I just might bash her head in with the way she treats Millie. I've seen her throw Millie in a chair and Millie says she does the same thing when she puts her to bed. Everything, done with force.

Why do they put news on? All it does is depress us. Although I have to admit this one made almost made sense.

A doctor reported: Alzheimer's may 'not' be a dementia, because it deals with plaques and tangles.

Sometimes they cause dementia and at times they don't cause dementia.

Different from TIA's, or Multi infarct, stroke dementia.

I found this very interesting. So, maybe Alzheimer's *is* in a class by itself. *Um, a disease all its own.*

But I really wish they'd put on cartoons, that would make us laugh.

I sit next to Millie, thinking if Blondie lays one more hand on her, she's gone.

I get the feeling Millie's reading my mind. Usually the only time we're able to read minds is when we face each other with our eyes. That connection, as Rose and I had. But thinking of Blondie and getting rid of her, I have the feeling Millie knows, especially when I get her approval with a smile.

Then I see Blondie near the nurse's station, clocking in. Good, she's on duty.

When Blondie came in my room after taking care of Millie, she proceeded to comb her blond mane in front of the bathroom mirror.

I sat on the bed looking out the window, thinking, how are we going to do this? What happens if she doesn't take the sip?

I had gotten an opened can of Mountain Dew soda from Brain's nephew. Don't like the stuff myself. Had it years ago coming back from the research center with Rose, and threw most of it out. Rose had gotten fast heart beats and wound up in the hospital.

Now a can sits on my dresser.

After combing her hair in the bathroom, she came to me with that flare she has, bouncing around as if she's a Broadway star, doing the last act of Gypsy.

"Well, hello Carol, and how are you?" she asked.

I looked at her, "Rata, rata, rata," *I don't care for the way you're treating Millie.*

"I see you are your usual self. Okay, it's sleepy sleep time so let's get dressed." and walked toward the dresser, opening the middle drawer taking out my pajamas. "Oh, what's this?" she asked, holding the can of Mountain Dew.

"rata, rata" *for you,* I said.

"Maybe later."

Bending down taking my shoes off I want to kick her and send her clear across the room. I want to smack her, pound her into the ground, but I sit letting her do her thing. Shoes, socks, then slacks. Bottom pjs on, then Lilly blouse and bra, replaced by blue. I always liked my light blue silk pajamas with a dark blue stipe on cuffs, pants and top. Silk made it easier moving around in bed from side to side or back. No sticking to the sheets.

Now dressed, she wants me in the bathroom to wash. Doesn't it go the other way, wash then dress? She takes my hand and leads me. I stop at the dresser near the soda can. *Sure you don't want a drink now?*

But she doesn't read minds like my friends.

She pulls harder at my arm and I follow, not wanting to upset her.

On the pot I pee, while she looks at herself in the mirror for the fiftieth time, tucking hair strands behind the ear, then in front. "Which looks best, front or back?" she asks, looking at me.

"Rata, rata rata …" *Frankly Blondie, I don't give a damn.*

"Same old saying. Carol, don't ever change your tune."

"Great, now your yelling has woken up the whole place."

I hear Ethel next door making noise, water running, potty seat banging, shower door slamming. And wonder what she's doing.

"You stay there," Blondie says, and leaves.

Meanwhile Ethel is having a grand ole time in her bathroom. She's gone poop and pee pee, and has scooped a handful of poop onto the wall.

She's become a wonderful finger painter with brown smears here and there. She's made brown clouds on the pale blue sky tile, also a few maple trees here and there, and was just getting into the grass when aide Blondie started yelling, "What the hell are you doing?"

And here Ethel thought she'd painted a beautiful picture for others to see. Only the cleaning crew got a chance to see Ethel's art work. Then pills were given and Ethel was in dream land.

Blondie came back, her hair a mess, and her face scrunched up as she's smelled something really bad.

I have new briefs that snap along the side, which should be easier to put on until I pushed my leg out making it harder for Blondie to adjust snaps.

"Come on Carol, move your leg so I can get these on. I had enough next door and don't need any more nonsense tonight."

"Rata, rata, rata," *not for you mommy dearest*, and push my leg out farther.

"Dammit Carol. Move your leg. I have a lot to do and you're not helping much."

I move my leg in and the brief goes on.

She takes a cloth with cold water and washes my face. Nothing I like better at night before going to bed then a cold wet cloth in my face. "RATA, RATA, RATA."

She grabs my hand.

I hold back.

"Would you please move your damn body and get into bed."

"Rata, Rata, Rata."

As we pass the soda can she stops.

Go ahead take a sip, Blondie.

"Oh what the hell," and flings me on the bed and grabs the can, drinking it all.

Now I can sleep peacefully. Millie doesn't know it yet, but she's gotten back at Blondie.

Around 1 a.m. doing bed checks, the new aide Ron, called for help.

Getting Blondie off the floor took some doing, while I was in never never land along with Ethel.

I knew that powered caffeine Brain's nephew left, would come in handy, especially after I mixed it in the Mountain Dew.

Bye bye Blondie.

Chapter 23

Today I got up as usual, had breakfast, listened to piano man, and blah, blah, blah, until the police came.

They questioned my friends, giving them a chance to tell their stories. The cop listened confused then asked again in a slow, deliberate voice, "Now ... tell me again ... what happened to aide Darlene ... and the blonde one?"

Again, my friends told the officer what they thought. When he asked me I told him the same, just a little different, "Sha, sha, sha ... Rata, rata, rata." I told him how the aides threw us around and were mean to us. But he kept shaking his head, and then asked to use the phone to call his superior.

"Sir, I don't think we have anything to go on here," he said. "It looks like a dead end."

And that was it.

After the police left, I thanked Josephine, Millie, and a few others for throwing the cops off.

'Too bad he didn't speak our language,' Josephine said, and we all laughed.

Then Jennifer came showing pictures of her family. "See how tall my daughter is. She's sixteen, almost as tall as me. Do you believe that?" I looked at the pictures, which were nice, but I wanted time to myself. I wanted a way out. I wanted the homeless camp back.

When Jennifer led me back to my room, I knew it was either potty or nap time. They treat us like children. And I'm not a child. I wonder why some treat us as children and others treat us as if we don't know anything. Like we're insane. Yes, that's the word, insane.

I haven't known many insane people in my life, maybe one, when growing up. A neighbor. She was nice and then all of a sudden she acted odd. She yelled at anyone who walked pasted her house, the paper boy, even the milk man. I didn't understand, because if it weren't for them she wouldn't have the paper to read or milk to drink. She should have realized that. But Mother told me, stay away from Mrs. Hingelstine. Mom said she'd gone through a bad time when she lost her husband in the war, and now old memories were coming back to 'haunt her'. Mom's word, haunt. I wondered if it were like ghosts coming in the middle of the night haunting children? Maybe Mr. Hingelstine was coming back to say hello to his wife, or get back at her for treating him badly. But she didn't really treat him badly. She told him what to do, like mow the lawn, throw the garbage out, wash the windows. Things a husband did around the house. Maybe she didn't say it in a nice way and that's why he came back to haunt her.

I didn't pay much attention because I was busy riding my bike or jumping rope with my friends.

But I notice some aides treat us, me, as if I'm insane. I wonder why those at the homeless camp didn't. They understood me and I understood them. Not all, but some. I wish I could speak the aides' language. I'd give them a word or two. I guess like Mrs. Hingelstine gave us kids. Maybe I am no different than Mrs. Hingelstine.

After Jennifer left, I waited a few minutes, then got up. Looking down the hall towards the nurse's station, I saw her yacking with others. I made my way around the corner and headed to John's room, down the other hall.

Five people are at the end of this hall. 'The dying corner', we call it. But John? He was healthy when I last saw him.

I'll open his door and when he sees me he'll be happy. I just know it.

Carol slowly opens the door and blinks, *this can't be John.* He's so thin. He's part of the mattress.

She moves closer. His eyes are closed and he's connected to a breathing machine and a nose tube. *Oxygen...* she thinks. He looks ten years older. How could it be? I was only homeless a short time.

After collecting herself she says, *Hi John*, even though his eyes are closed. She sits on his bed, close to him. *Hello John, what's happening?* No answer, but she sees his eye lids flutter.

Seen any good looking women lately? And she waits for a smile, but none comes.

John, what happened? How did you get so ill?

His eyes open and she sees the smile in them. He doesn't need to speak. She knows he recognizes her and is happy she's come to visit.

What happened, John? she asks.

Too much medication. When I wouldn't take pills they gave me shots. I had no choice. I couldn't fight them, there were too many.

Who did this John? Carol asks.

One of our favorites, Marissa.

Carol remembers. *Marissa was next on her list before she went to the homeless camp.*

She spends the rest of the visit telling John about the homeless camp, how nice it was. *I wish we could make our own camp away from this place.*

John agrees.

***

In the corner of the television room Carol talks with her friends, *Who's on Medicaid?* she asks. Almost all answer, *I am. I am.*

When you live in a nursing home and run out of money, there's a look back period of three years. Most of my friends are on Medicaid, a few waiting to spend their money down, or give it to relatives, not having a husband or wife become destitute. I wonder if they had gotten divorced, prior to look back, if it would have made a difference. Then they'd each have their own money.

Carol tells them she's not on Medicaid yet. Rose pays her bills. But knows the money won't last forever. It's too expensive living here. What then? Medicaid. Then she'd be like everyone else, poor and on government help, which doesn't give much these days. And what happens when the government runs out of money because they gave it to other countries to help fight *their* wars. What happens when there's no money?

Carol never wanted to be dependent on anyone, especially Rose, or the government. She wanted to care for herself. She was strong. But it's impossible to pay thousands every month and not go broke.

She wonders what people in other countries do? Do they have universal health care? Was it good? Did it pay for all a person's needs?

She was the one who cared for her mother, until she put her mother in a nursing home. And now the same is happening to her. She doesn't want to wind up on the dying corner.

Chapter 24

I put pills from my little pouch in Marissa's cup of coffee that she left on my table. She'd gone to clean up the bathroom and get new briefs for me from the hall closet. When back, she picked up her cup and drank.

I waited for her to go down, the way Fatso did, but she didn't. It took longer. Maybe because Marissa was younger, not fat, in better shape. Don't know the reason, all I know is I stood by the door and waited. She came toward me, eyes full of hatred, which I didn't blame her for. But quickly forgot, when I remembered how she wiped my behind, and other areas on my body with such force that led to skin wounds and infections. And, I didn't forget how she treated John.

Her fisted hand swiped at me. I sucked in. She missed, falling, hitting her head on the door knob and her arm wrapped behind her. She tried getting up three times, then lay still.

I waited, making sure it was done. Minutes later I slipped out of my room, closing the door.

Walking down the hall I saw the two teenage abusive aides. *Um, they're still on my list.* I haven't forgotten the abuse they gave Sophie, and god knows who else.

"Rata, rata, rata," I said.

They look at me. "Oh, she's nuts," one said. "Do you really think so?" the other asked.

"Yeah, she has no idea what's going on. All she does is walk the halls and talk, her talk, to others here."

"Do you think they understand each other?"

"No way. Did you ever hear them? They sound like a bunch of chattering monkeys."

"RATA, RATA, RATA," *hey little girls who are you abusing today?* I asked, in my monkey chatter.

"You sure she doesn't understand we're talking about her?"

"I tell you, she's nuts."

"RATA. RATA. RATA." *Come. Follow. Me.* I repeat and they start after me. Good, they heard me, or mind to mind connection. I lead them to my room, not opening the door, but knocking on it.

"See, I told you she's nuts," One says. "She's knocking on her own door."

Inside, I'd left the television on loud.

"We should turn the TV off if she's out here," the other says.

I left them and went to the dining room where my friends were getting ready for dinner. Just as I entered the dining room I heard two teenage girls yell, "Holy Shit. What the heck happen to Marissa?"

It turned out two teenage volunteer aides, decided not to come to work anymore, because they didn't enjoy seeing bodies mutilated, heads bashed in, bleeding, and arms twisted out of sockets.

Bucket list complete.

Chapter 25

Rose saw the news this morning and didn't like it. She doesn't like most news but this story bothered her a lot.

A man, husband to his Alzheimer's wife, is on trial for rape. Raping his wife, that is, in an Alzheimer's unit. The end of life unit.

The aides saw him visit his wife, close the door, then lock it. When listening by the door, they heard noises. Then half an hour or less the husband came out and left the facility.

It seems when the aides went to check his wife, she was wet, down at her privates. Later testing showed semen. Husband's semen.

The rape trial went on for weeks, and then in the end he was acquitted.

I wondered, suppose this was Carol's room, would it be rape then, being she wasn't the man's wife?

My thoughts went to this wife who knew nothing, being in later stage of Alzheimer's. And she wasn't being abused? What a joke. It turned out; all men were on the jury.

Rose gets call after call from the nursing home, "Carol is missing." "Carol is causing a disturbance."

Why can't Carol have docile dementia, like others Rose has seen at the nursing home? Why does she have to upset everyone?

Too bad Rose doesn't know the happiness Carol's brought, Sally, Marti, Stanley, Brain and John, especially Millie. Too bad Rose doesn't know the calmness Carol gives Millie, makes Millie feel alive, not dead, sitting slumped over, drugged, in a wheelchair day after day. Too bad.

After another doctor's visit, Rose went to visit Carol. She feels well enough to take on anything Carol is doing or has done.

When she gets there, she's met with Head of Nursing, who tells her about Marissa and the teenage volunteers. "Carol is very upset losing her favorite aide, Marissa," says head of nursing. And Rose thinks, *I'll go to her right now, take her for ice cream. That'll make her feel better.*

She finds Carol in the television room, talking her talk to others, thinking, *they have to be annoyed with Carol.* But she notices something. She sees the others listening to Carol, their eyes wide open, and wonders, *do they understand each other?*

"Hi Ca," Rose says, "Let's go for chocolate ice cream. Okay?"

She almost waits for an answer, but Carol looks sad, and should be, losing one of her aides. Little does she know Carol's sad for John and what they've done to him.

"C'mon Ca, let's go. Sorry folks we're going downstairs," as she looks at the others, and takes Carol's hand.

Carol's other hand latches onto Millie's wheelchair, *I'll be back,* she says, *I promise.*

Everyone understands, except Rose.

They go for ice cream, and Rose walks Carol outside, as usual. Then go to *their* bench, the one that overlooks the pond where fish jump. An Anhinga is in the middle of the water on the pump, airing his wings out, after diving for his lunch.

Carol likes Anhinga's, and most birds, but her favorite is the Red Cardinal, she's always called Geech. Rose wonders if Carol remembers when they saw Geech at the condo, and fed him, his wife, Geechetta, and his children. Rose often thinks of those times with lightheartedness. Those were good times. These times, Rose doesn't understand why any of this happened.

Why Carol got sick with this horrific disease, Alzheimer's? It's worse than being dead. In fact, it would be better if Carol were dead than to see her like this. So different. Agitated all the time. So crazy. She wonders what they'd be doing if Carol weren't ill. Would they be playing golf? Walking the heart trail, playing tennis, riding bikes to the beach, then for a swim in the beautiful warm salt water? Then home to take showers and have a drink on the patio with neighbors or alone? It was always fun being around Carol. She had something interesting to say all the time. Information on every subject: stock markets, golf, weather, travel, animals—her favorite. How could one person change so much?

Carol tried telling Rose all that had gone on, Marissa, and the teenage aides, but Rose didn't listen. She never did.

After their walk around the pond Carol knows it's time for Rose to leave. It always happens that way.

They go upstairs and Rose kisses her on the cheek, and puff, she's gone. But that's okay this time, because Carol has other things to do.

***

Patients sleep with mouths wide open, some snoring. I see the nurse with long brown hair squirt hot sauce in their mouths. Why? What's the purpose? But then I look at the clock. It's late, time for nurse to go home. I'm sure she wants folks awake, so she can hand out her meds.

I watch Josephine, cough, and spit out what the nurse has put in her mouth. She hasn't done it to me, yet. Guess because I don't sleep much, and when they give me pills I hide them in my pouch.

Josephine starts yelling, and nurse has the meds right there ready for her take. Then Josephine can sleep and nurse can go home.

Great way to run a nursing home.

Chapter 26

Getting off the escalator in the basement, Carol inches along the wall, listening for voices and hears none. She bypasses the room she'd gone into before, leading her further down a dark hall.

In the dark she squints, ears open for anything. Nothing. She notices another door, dark in color, almost black, without a handle. She pushes and it slightly opens. She pushes more seeing the contents. They have more rooms in this place then anyone knows. What is this room for?

High metal tables face her. Skinny tables, maybe twenty or more. Wonder what *they're* for?

All but three are covered with white flat sheets. She lifts one sheet, nothing, cold hard table underneath. She goes to the lumpy-sheet one and lifts the sheet then steps back. Staring at her is a dead person, Who? A friend? A closer look she sees the body doesn't fill the table. *Half a body?* She pulls the sheet back. *Not even half. Head, shoulders and chest, that's it. Do I know this person?*

She hears noise outside the door and ducks under an empty table.

Two men enter. Workmen, she presumes, ready to paint something. One has paint splotches on his sleeve. She pulls the sheet on the table down farther hiding her crouching body. He takes a tool from his jumpsuit-waist-loop and scrapes the face of the person on the table. She wants to say, *Hey, stop. You're hurting the person.* But she doesn't. Those words are no longer a part of her. She wants to yell, but holds her voice. The other man takes leftover scraps and puts them in a rag. He scrapes and scrapes and she hears the other guy say, "So you gonna make this one blonde? When you get done she'll be beautiful."

The scraper answers, "I'm not sure what they want us to do with this one. At least the one over there is a guy, that's easy. Short hair or bald. Maybe mustache, depends if it fits the guy in #303"

303? Mikes room, Carol thinks. He has a mustache some times, depending on who shaves him. Some aides are lazy and don't shave the men, but Jennifer shaves and cuts his hair making him look like he's just come from the barber. *Why are they making half a body to look like Mike?* He's been here a long time—one of the longest.

"They'll never miss him once we get through with him," the scraper says. "With the recording, no one will ever know."

What do they mean? 'Recordings?

"Okay Tony, I think that's it for now. I'll have to work on the eyes a bit more. They look fake, don't ya think?"

"Yeah. Maybe more lashes on the bottom. Remember he's Italian. They have thick lashes."

"You're right, that's what I'm missing. Tomorrow though, not now. Then he'll be ready for the weekend. C'mon, let's clock out and get something to drink."

"Gotcha. You're turn to buy."

Cleaning up, they argued who was buying beers.

Carol's knees hurt when she tried standing. Crouched in the same position too long, she's not as young as she used to be.

She passes Mike's twin, wondering what they're going to do with it. Thinking, wait till Brain hears this. He thinks the room with stinky rotten food boxes was big? Wait'ill he hears Mike has a double.

She winds up in the television room wanting to tell everyone she sees, but the news is on and everyone's listening, even aides.

Some news she can't believe, then again after what she's seen and done, most doesn't surprise her.

'A 62 year old woman went missing, wandered off, right around a full moon. When they found her she was dead in the woods.'

'76 year old man went missing, but was found safe later.'

That's a good story, she thought. But then the announcer said, 'the man couldn't say where he'd been, because he spoke another language.' And she thought, *why didn't they have him talk to us.*

The next news story told of an 'Elderly couple with dementia missing from assisted living facility.' And she wondered, *was one helping the other find their way Home.*

Then a '72 year old woman missing. They found her, but she died two days later in hospital.' *I guess they didn't find her soon enough.*

The worse story, 'In Japan, ten thousand dementia people go missing each year.'

Were they all looking for Home? She wonders.

Imagine if the news heard her stories.

Chapter 27

I'm walking, fall over a person in the hall I didn't see. I get up and try helping the woman up, but she doesn't want help, so I continue on. I need to get out of here.

Millie's further down the hall, waiting for an aide to wash and dress her for bed. She calls to me with her eyes, *Did you hear about Josephine?*

I ask in my voice, "Sha. Sha sha?" *No. What happened?*

She found the way out I told you about, and wound up in the pond. She yelled loud and someone jumped in and saved her, Millie says.

No kidding. I wonder how many others know that way out.

Don't know, I haven't asked anyone else. Anyway, they found her and put her in lock-down. They locked her in her room. Do you believe that?

Poor Josephine, I bet she could use some company. Maybe we can visit her, I say.

Sure if you can figure out how to unlock her door.

Oh, I'll have to work on that one. Picking locks is not my forte, although I've done pretty well so far.

***

Passing Mike's room Carol sees him in bed. She knocks softly, but no one says come in. She enters the room seeing Mike's closed eyes. *He must be really sick.*

"Sha Sha, sha?" *Hi Mike, what's the matter? We missed you at breakfast?*

No answer.

Mike, You okay?

Nothing.

She touches his cheek, hoping to wake him. "Sha … sha, sha." *Mike … time to get up.*

Nothing.

He doesn't feel like he has a fever, she thinks. In fact he feels cool.

Maybe he stayed up too late last night. Yeah, that's probably it. I'll come back later, when he's awake.

She closes the door so no one else will bother him.

***

Another television news story: A 51 year old employee of a nursing home is accused of beating a

77 year old patient who suffers from Alzheimer's disease. She was arrested and charged with injury to an elder.

Police said she was caught on a hidden camera in the victim's room. The victim has been a patient for a year at the facility. Police said the daughter put a hidden camera in her mother's room because she always had unexplained injuries. The hidden camera showed the aide hitting the older woman in the face, and then threw her on the bed. The camera also showed the patient being pulled up by her arm, with force.

It happens all the time here, maybe not as much anymore, being some abusers have gone to heaven or hell.

Chapter 28

Vivian came to see me today. She told me she's quitting her job. "I like the people Carol, but I don't like the way they treat their patients. Most aides don't care about their work at all. It's just a job to them. The money isn't good, so I don't know why they stay in health care."

"Sha, sha, sha," *I don't know either.* Thinking maybe Vivian understood me. I felt at times she did, especially when she walked the halls with me on her break. I tried telling her she was different. She was one of the good ones that others could learn from. I hope I see her again.

***

After dinner, Carol visits Mike and finds him sitting up in bed with eyes wide open.

"Sha, Sha," *Hi Mike I see you're feeling better.* He nods.

"Sha, sha, sha." *I'm glad. When I saw you this morning, you really looked bad. I figured you stayed up to late last night. Did you eat dinner?*

Mike shakes his head, saying, "No."

She looks at him and asks, "Sha sha sha?" *Are you hungry? Can I get you something?*

He shakes his head again.

"Oh, okay. I thought I'd get you something. I have bread and peanut butter in my dresser. Sure you don't want *something*?"

He shakes his head, and says, "No."

"Sha sha sha sha," *Sounds like you have a cold. You sure you're okay?*

Again, shakes his head.

"Sha sha sha," *Think you'll be at breakfast tomorrow?* Carol asks.

He Nods, saying, "Yes."

An aide comes in, "Carol, what are you doing here?"

"Rata, rata, rata." *Mike is sick. Something's wrong with him.*

"Okay Carol, you have to leave now. Let Mike get his rest." And the aide pushes her to the door.

Passing Mike's legs, Carol sees a flat-bed under the sheet and blanket but doesn't think any more of it.

She tells the others, *Mike is ill. He doesn't sound right. Something's wrong.*

***

Downstairs again, she doesn't see Mikes' double, but sees others. All are half bodies.
What's going on?

***

Back in Mike's room I pull his bed sheet back, nothing. No legs. No feet. Nothing. Only half a body.

Why would they cut his body in half? For what reason?

Are others like this?

A closer inspection shows me this is not the real Mike. It's a dummy, made to look like him. I touch his head, hard. He was always hardheaded but not this hard. The dummy has a wig. Mike never wore wigs. He said, 'a person should grow old with dignity, look like themselves, the way God intended.'

His face is made of a hard material. *Ah ha*, the carving man downstairs, while the other guy wiped up shavings. They were working on a woman, if I remember correctly.

"Sha, Sha." *Hi Mike*, I say.

Imitation Mike's says, "Hi."

"Sha sha sha?" *How are you?* I ask.

"Yes," he answers.

"Sha sha sha sha? *What are you going to do today?* I ask.

One answer back, "Yes."

Apparently half-body Mike is set for one word answers, not conversations. Anyone would think this is a real Mike. I'm glad it's not, but where is the real Mike?

I straighten the covers and place imitation Mike's head back on the pillow, the way it was, and leave. I have a job to do.

I go to the dying corner. Who else is new? I have to find out what's going on with my friends.

I've already lost Sally. What about John? He's ill. I have to keep an eye on John.

***

Carol and Brian figure the nursing home is making half bodies of those who have died, or helping others on Medicaid to die. They put them on the dying wing, using voice recordings, so others think they're still alive. When Medicaid does name checks, the names are still in the home's records, but in half body form. And home gets paid.

Carol is caught giving pills to the man with glasses who stares at her in the dining room. She's tried helping him, but he started hitting her.

She felt sorry for him, and his wife, who came to see him every other day. One day the wife didn't come and Carol saw how sad he was, either lying in bed or slumped over in his wheelchair, so why not give *him* peace, she thought. His wife would probably die before him, being she was sick when she came, but that wasn't happening. Carol gave him her pouch pills and within minutes it was over.

Later she saw people in front of his door, wheeling a covered body out. She was thankful he didn't become half a body, like others.

Apparently the wife had placed a camera in an empty book that lay on the night stand. But the nursing home did nothing about it, being it would be placed under investigation, which they didn't want.

***

In the television room Carol sees no one's playing the piano. A visitor decides to talk about her mother.

"I went in my mother's room and she was sound asleep. Her arms and head were resting on the table over the bed. She should have been in bed lying down, or sitting in a chair."

I looked at the lady next to me, saying with our eyes, *so what's new about that? We do it all the time.*

The woman went on saying things were not right. She saw lots of problems with the food, and keeping patients locked up.

Again, *what's new with that? That's the way it is and has been since I got here.*

One resident spoke up saying she'd written a letter but was afraid to send it, thinking she'd be thrown out and be homeless.

My thoughts. *It's better being homeless than here. I know. I was at a homeless camp.*

The woman talking about her mother says, "You know, it's up to all of you to change the system.

You have to write letters to the government, and people who own this place. Tell them what your dislikes are. Only you can change it, no one else."

I thought, *how can I change it? I can't speak the words health care speaks. How can I possibly change it? Sure those who speak words like the aides, nurses and Rose, can change it. But how could I, or we, change it?* I look at Millie, who agrees.

The only way would be to get someone to write for us. Vivian came to mind. She didn't like it here because they treated patients bad. She understood me at times, especially when we spent time together. She was able to connect with my eyes and know what was in my head. Maybe Vivian can send letters to the owners for us. Tell them we know how their defrauding Medicaid with half-bodies. Tell them about aides who are nasty, and others I easily got rid of. Wait a minute that would get me in trouble, and I'd wind up in jail.

Vivian gave me her number in case of emergency, but how can I phone her? Maybe I can ask Brian, he understands both languages. He can tell her I want to see her. Yes, I'll ask my buddy, Brian.

Chapter 29

I'm walking and fall over a person who has their legs up in that bed-type chair. I try to get up. I can't. *Oooh, pain, bad in my side.* I try again, pain screams through my body. What happened? Again I try, and my leg falls out from underneath me. I can't get off the floor. People come, with a wheelchair. "Rata, Rata, Rata, Rata" *No, I don't want to get in that.* Don't they hear me?

The girl who stays with me is sitting in the blue-drape room watching TV soap operas. I don't like them. I'm wheeled next to the bed. I try to get up. *Oh, it hurts,* and sit back down.

Hours later, Rose comes, kisses me on the forehead. *Where have you been?* I ask in my words. *I've been calling you for hours.*

She says hello to me and the girl. I don't know why the girl is here, she doesn't walk with me down the hall for my way out of here. Good though, Rose is here, she'll get me out of this place.

"What's the matter, Ca? Why aren't you up walking the halls?" Rose asks.

Can't you see I'm in pain? That's why. The girl and Rose talk, then she leaves. She comes back with a woman dressed in white. Minutes later they're taking me through the doors that slide back. Fire Engine blares, Rose does that thing near the door and the blaring stops. The doors come together. We're in that small room, moving. Then the doors slide back, and Rose wheels me fast down another hall. She talks to someone who meets us. X-ray, the sign on the door reads. I'm put on a cold, hard table. "Rata. Rata. Rata." *OH. IT. HURTS.* Rose has her hand on my cheek, saying. "It's okay Ca, I promise we will go for chocalotta ice cream after this." I love chocalotta anything. My name for chocolate, not hers, I made up years ago. She used to laugh a lot, she doesn't anymore. I still think she's ill?

There's a machine over me on the table. It hurts so bad. Why can't they help me? This table is hard. The man comes back and talks to Rose. Something's broken, he says. Rose is upset, crying, "What do I do now?" she says. My God what is it that's so bad that makes her cry? She never cried, only when I pushed her out of the shower, and they told her I had some 'A' disease.

Next I'm lying on a soft bed in a truck/car. Rose isn't with me. She stayed at that place. 'Hospital' the man tells me. Oh Boy, Rose must be sick and they're taking me to her. That's it. But I wish my leg would stop hurting.

"Rata Rata Rata Rata." *Why are you doing this?* I yell at the woman tying ropes on my wrists. She leaves. I can't move my arms. I yell, "Rata, Rata …" but no one hears.

Thank God, Rose comes, says hello and kisses me on the forehead. When she sees my hands tied to the bed, she says, "Be right back, Ca." In the hall I hear her tell someone, "Please untie her." And the person answers, "She can't get up." Rose answers, "She won't." Rose comes and unties my hands. I try sitting up, wanting out of this confusion. Rose pushes me back down, "No Ca, you can't get up."

I stay.

Soon I'm in another room and Rose sits by my side. She won't leave me, I know. 'Be at your side', the pictures inscription that I gave her long ago. 'Don't walk in front of me I may not lead, Don't walk behind me I may not follow, Just walk beside me and be my friend.' I remember when I found it in my closet many years ago, and knew then that I wanted to give it to Rose. She worried too much. I thought this inscription would make her stop worrying and live life as it came. As I did.

Much later I sleep, and then see large white lights and people with masks dressed in blue all around me. I sleep more.

When I wake Rose is at my side. Good.

She stays, until I'm brought back to the four story place where I walk the halls. I want to walk again, but they won't let me. They put me in a wooden box and call it therapy, saying, "You have to learn to stand before you can walk." Standing long makes me tired and I fall asleep.

Rose comes often, but most of the time I don't know she's here because I sleep a lot. Why have they done this to me?

Finally in a wheelchair I sit day after day, like Millie, until it's time for bed. I try to get up and someone yells, 'sit back down'. Why won't they let me walk?

I stand, and fall, after my first step. They pick me up and put me in the chair. "DON'T GET UP, CAROL," they yell. I stay seated.

***

On this day I stand from the chair. What do I do now? How can I go forward? Nothing moves. I move my hips, nothing. My feet won't move, how do I move them? I'll try harder. Finally they move and my knee, shoulder and arm hit the floor.

Rose comes. "What happened? You're full of bruises."

"Sha, sha, sha, sha," *I tried to walk and fell*. But Rose doesn't listen. She's mad, and rolls me to the desk where the women in white and bug-shirt people are.

"Does she need to fall out of the chair and break something else," she yells. "Can't you put something on the chair to stop her from falling?"

"No," bug-shirt aide says. "It's against the rules. Patients' rights. No restraints."

Rose's mad, shakes her head, "Rules are meant to be broken, you know."

She wheels me away, and finally we're with the ice cream lady. *Yay*, about time. I haven't had my favorite in a long time. She has cups of ice cream in her hand and pushes me forward to our tree, where we watch ducks in the pond, and flutterbys come to say hello. Flutterbys are so beautiful.

Yummy, so good. I love chocalotta ice cream. I can't get enough into my mouth. Rose gives me small amounts on the tip of the spoon and sings to me. We have fun under the shade tree. People further away are having fun. But Rose and I are together enjoying ice cream.

The drugs they're giving me won't let me hold my eyes open, but every so often I open them, catching a glimpse of Rose looking at me. She looks sad.

Why can't we go home? Why do we have to stay here? Home I can see you every day, here I can't.

"Wow, Carol did you see that fish jump?" Rose asks. But I didn't. My eyes were closed, and I was in that other place I go some times.

It's not a bad place. In fact, it's kind of nice, calm and quiet. There's a beauty there that's hard to describe. The colors are vibrant, and the music, violins mostly, soothing. Folks come and go as they please, not like here, where you can't get up and go where you want. This other place is heavenly.

Oops, here we go. Rose is making cross blessings on my forehead. Guess she's leaving soon. Yep, now we're headed to sliding door room. And there's a bug-shirt lady. Here we go again. One nice thing, Rose puts me in front of the bird cage. It stands around ten feet tall and holds at least ten birds. I see the birds on the floor of the cage even if I can't lift my head. They sing me to sleep most times.

"God bless you Ca," she says, and kisses my forehead. She's nice. I like her. She walks to the retractable door room, and is gone.

Bye Rose.

Chapter 30

In the afternoon new bug-shirt people are on duty. One I can't stand is here, and wonder why she can't be like Vivian.

"Okay Carol, let's go to the bathroom," she says, and wheels me down the end of the hall. *There's that door, pasted the Exit sign, near the window. Some day, maybe.*

Bug-lady lifts under my arms and puts me on the toilet. "Now pee pee," she says.

"Rata, rata, rata," *You do pee pee yourself.*

She leaves, and I'm left alone.

Oh, I hurt. My legs are numb. Can't someone take me off here? The door is open and I see the clock on the other wall reads four o'clock. I've been on this seat half an hour. Why do they leave me so long until I can't feel my legs or feet? "Rata, Rata, Rata, Rata." *Is anyone there?*

Eyes close. I'm in that other place, the quiet place. I see a woman sitting at a stream, running her hand through flowing water, enjoying the sunshine. A dog with long hair runs around, not barking, just running, having fun with birds that have landed and taken off in front of him. He wags his tail in a friendly way.

"RATA, RATA, RATA" *Get me off this pot! Where are you? I'm numb, my back hurts. Get me off here. Please.*

The bug-lady comes. "Good girl, you did pee pee," she says, then struggles putting on a brief.

"Sha, Sha, Sha, Sha" *Why didn't you come sooner?*

Bug-lady pulls my pants up then throws me in the chair making it hit the wall. We are off to the dining room.

When seated at the dining table she puts the brakes on. More people come, three others placed at the table.

I know Margaret, she's nice. *High Peggy*, she likes when I call her that.

The other two people I don't know. *Hi, nice to see you,* I say. But no one answers except Peggy, *Nice to see you Carol. Where you been?*

"Sha, sha, sha ..." *I went outside. My friend, Rose, came and we had ice cream.*

Oh, that's nice. No one comes to see me anymore. My children live out of state, come only in the winter, once a year. You're lucky to have a loved one close by.

Yes, I am lucky to have Rose. She's nice, but I feel sorry for her.

At that, bug-shirt lady sits next to Peggy and starts stuffing potatoes in her mouth. I guess I'm next. The other two sit, with eyes half closed.

***

All my friends are gone, or have become half bodies. Even Millie, the first person I met in the dining room. The first person I could talk to, who understood me. Out of all my friends she was the one who didn't question me getting out of this place. I'm sure if she didn't have that wheelchair she would have joined me.

It amazes me how much people talk. Even when they don't have anything to say. They talk and talk, words come out of their mouth saying nothing. I think they like to hear their own voice. That's my own opinion.

Most of the time you don't need to talk much at all, especially if you know the person. All you need to do is look them in the eyes and they understand with one word or two.

Like Mille and I, we spoke little sound with our mouth, but we understood each other with our eyes. Millie couldn't make many sounds, except laugh or cry. I'm glad I made her laugh.

I miss my friend.

***

Am I afraid to die? In a way, yes. Then in a way, no. I know if there's no reason to live, then I want to die. I think. But then there's always a glimpse, a thought, something will change, and make me want to live. What is that something?

I'd like to be well again, outside playing golf with Rose. Playing tennis. Soaking up sun rays and seeing that beautiful blue-green ocean I love so much, out having a martini before dinner, talking with my friend. So many things I'd like to live for.

Is it going to change now? Is this one 'Word disease' going to leave me?

Chapter 31

Rose hasn't been well and is afraid to drive: feeling dizzy, brain fog, off balance and other disturbing physical and mental feelings.

She went to a new doctor today, a specialist. Her general practitioner and another doctor suggested she see a neurologist.

Nervous, knowing something was wrong other than high blood pressure, she filled out the form for the new doctor. Feeling as though there were fog, or large cloud in her brain, she filled the questions out to the best to her ability. She got name, address, phone number, mother's name, father's name, siblings. Then the questions started: what's wrong? After twenty minutes, she'd filled out what she could when her name was called.

She followed the very young woman into an office. "Doctor will be right with you," the woman said.

She sat waiting, going over the short notes she'd made so she wouldn't have to try and remember what she's been feeling. She wasn't happy being here, and wanted to go home but she also knew something was wrong.

Especially in her brain.

Too many times she became disoriented, confused as to the time of day or where she was. Many times she stared out the living room window thinking, it's ten o'clock in the morning, only to look at the clock on her computer reading three o'clock in the afternoon.

Then she heard high heels in the hallway and the door opened. "Good morning," the woman in a white short coat said, with her hand out stretched toward Rose.

Rose shook the doctor's hand, and watched her sit across from her at a computer.

The doctor did some typing then questioned, "So, what brings you here today?"

Rose looked at her notes. "I don't like the way I've been feeling."

"Oh. What are you feeling?"

"At times I feel I'm losing my mind." There she said it.

"I see you've had a heart attack and have high blood pressure. Does it run in the family?" asked the doctor.

Rose answered, yes to heart disease and cancer running in her family. "But no one had brain illness." She didn't mention Carol, the dear friend, the second family. She wanted to, but didn't think it necessary.

After all, the doctor wanted blood relatives.

"Why do you think you're losing your mind?"

Rose went into the confusion to time of day, not remembering what day it was, seeing faces she knew but couldn't remember their names. Just a familiar face.

"Okay, I'm going to give you three words to remember, Camel, Rainbow, and Football."

Rose repeated the three words, "Camel, Rainbow, Football."

"I'm going to ask you to repeat them in a few minutes, but first I'd like you to draw a clock," and the doctor handed Rose a sheet of paper.

"You want me to draw a clock? With hands, or without?"

"I want the time reading 2:50, so yes, hands on the clock."

Rose drew a circle, and then wrote 12, 3, 6, 9 in their rightful place. She put a dot in the middle of the circle and started to draw hands, but couldn't remember how to. There was no 2 or 50.

She thought hard, then said, "This is stupid. Don't you have a different test?"

"Take your time. There's no rush." And the doctor typed in her computer.

Rose thought hard, not coming up with numbers between 12 and 3, or 3 to 6 or other in between numbers.

She didn't use this type of clock anymore. All the clocks in the house were digital lights. Only one circle clock was on the book shelf in the dining room, which she never looked at. Now she wished she had it here. At one point she looked on the four walls to see if there was a hanging clock, but none to be found.

Then Rose remembered when Carol went to the doctor and he'd given her the same test. Carol had passed it, drew the clock and remembered three words.

What were those three words she's supposed to remember? Rainbow, one, she remembered that one. What were the other two? Football, her ex played football. One left. It wouldn't come and her brain felt on overload.

"Okay, time's up," the doctor said, interrupting her jumbled thoughts.

"Crazy. I just couldn't draw a clock. I don't believe it. How stupid."

"No problem, sometimes that happens. Can you repeat the three words I mentioned before.

"Rainbow, Football, ... Uh ..." She closed her eyes in deep thought trying to remember the last word, finally saying, "I can't remember." Amazed she couldn't remember, she finally asked, "What was it?"

"Camel," the doctor said, and Rose thought of cigarettes she smoked years ago, but she couldn't remember the word today.

"I'm giving you a script for blood work to be done this week, and there's a cup in the bathroom for a urine sample. I'll meet you at the front desk."

Rose gathered her herself, still upset not remembering words and clock numbers. Then went into the bathroom and peed in a cup.

She met the doctor at the front desk where she was handed a script for blood work. Then paid what Medicare didn't, and left.

On the drive home she thought: What is it like to have dementia?

Just a word? No. Dementia isn't even a word. It shouldn't qualify as anything, especially a word. Words mean something, This is a devastating word, a word that tears at you, thinking, it can't be. I can't have this word. No, not me! That happens to others, not me. That happened to Carol, it can't happen to me, too. What is the point to life, if in the long run we get this word? Nothing matters anymore. Nothing. I'm not only losing my memory, but feel awful everyday: confusion, nervous, disoriented, not finding the right word for a sentence. So many other things, besides losing your memory. Why don't people write about this, instead of just losing one's memory. I didn't tell the doctor there was more. Why don't they tell you what it's *really* like?

It took a while to get home, worrying at times if I were lost, when streets all looked the same.

I lay on the bed staring at the ceiling. Was the answer there? I stared and stared for hours, until the phone rang. I didn't answer. I didn't want to tell whoever it was I had Alzheimer's. No one should know. Just me and the doctor. No one else should know.

I lay thinking. Could I have Alzheimer's? I'll get another opinion. Another doctor. A smarter one. What do they know about Alzheimer's in a small town? What do they know? Period.

Here I was asking the same questions Carol must have asked herself.

How could it hit twice in one household?

When I first heard the word Alzheimer's a long time ago relating to Carol, it struck me as a lightening blot. How? Why? Where? How did she get it? Where did she get it? And, Why did she get it? I was in shock, not knowing what to do. How does one feel physically well, and then be told they have the hideous disease Alzheimer's?

Now I've thought of the word a second time, and it's pertaining to me *this* time. Me? Do I have Alzheimer's? Is this what Carol thought?

Sure, I had trouble finding right words for sentences. I couldn't even draw the face of a clock right. I got the circle, and 12, 3, 6, and 9. But couldn't figure what the numbers were in between.

I couldn't get my mind in order, the right order. It seemed all jumbled, out of sync. I was sure I had a dementia of some kind, possibly Alzheimer's. Little did I know there are so many different types of dementia. Maybe delirium should be listed under the Dementia category. Like in Chinese restaurants, column A, column B, and so on, different chicken dishes. Maybe Dementia is like a food, many different categories'.

It's *not* dementia, it's a urinary infection. A plain ordinary urinary infection. I've been put on antibiotics. By the sixth day I felt better, all feelings and thoughts I had were gone. I was 'me' again. In my right mind.

Fourteen days on antibiotic's and I was the old me. Able to walk the grocery store isles without dizziness, and all other symptoms.

I'm feeling better. I know what day it is. I don't feel confused or disoriented. Why didn't the first two doctors find this? No, I had to go to a neurologist to find I had a urinary infection and not dementia.

Chapter 32

Carol can't take living the way she is any more. She's tried getting out of the nursing home and failed. She always found herself back in the blue room, drugged then sleeping. Now, at wits end, she just can't take anymore.

She reaches her hand over the back of the headboard and grabs her pouch. She gathers all pills left in pouch, and adds the little left over caffeine powder into her bedside glass of water.

She's made amends with people she didn't like and forgave them for all they've done to hurt her. She didn't need to make amends with Rose, she still loved her and what she tried to do for her. But Rose will have to understand Carol's point of view—her hate for living without a mind. Never thinking she'd hate life, she takes the first sip.

Maybe she'll finally see her mother and father. Maybe things will be better. No, she knows they'll be better.

She takes another sip.

Good it's mid-morning. Aides are done working the floor, and everyone is napping, like her, or relaxing in the television room.

She wonders if anyone here will miss her. Maybe, but this is something she has to do for herself, and Rose.

She drinks the rest and lays back down. She closes her eyes, saying the prayers she remembers.

And that's that.

***

Today Rose feels the need for Carol. While at the kitchen window doing dishes, she looks out and cries, "Where are you? I need you Ca." She feels herself on the brink of crying, "I need you now, Ca. Where are you?" She looks to the sky, and there eye level, maybe six feet away, flies a red and brown Flutterby. It flies to the right, then turns, and flies back from where it came. She watches it in awe. *She heard me,* Rose thinks. Tears come. *She heard me.* There is something after Alzheimer's.

Chapter 33

Why didn't the nursing home tell me, Carol took those pills and killed herself? Why didn't they tell me? I wonder if they used her body for testing. Did they pull out her brain, dissect it into tiny little pieces?

It doesn't matter. In the end I cremated her, and gave her to the ocean. The blue-green water she loved so much. It doesn't really matter.

The nursing home finally was closed down after Brian spilled the story Carol had dictated to him. Good thing he spoke both languages.

The police were called in when government started checking on the dead. Looking into matters they found half bodies, and other interesting things in the basement with florescent lights. I'm glad they were closed, and wonder how many other facilities treat their patients as Carol, and others were treated.

Some workers feared the police due to their background working in other facilities.

Fatso's body left quickly when she was shoved into the furnace. Marissa's body was picked up by illegal immigrant relatives. Only Blondie's body was traced back to the orphanage she grew up in.

Chapter 34

I can see you Rose. You're as clear as the driven snow. You're my friend, my dear one, the one who took care of me, made sure 'they' took care of me. But you never knew how 'they' treated us. The abuse they gave us. They didn't care for us one bit. They only made it look like they were helping us when family and friends came to visit. Now you know the truth, and what really happened. I'm glad me and my friends were able to connect with each other.

Rose couldn't believe all she'd read. How could she not know all this was happening to Carol and others. Carol called them friends. So she really wasn't alone. She had others to talk to, who understood her.

Rose admired Carol for taking her own life. She doesn't think she, herself, could have done this. She'd thought many times how to make it easier on Carol by doing away with her, but she couldn't. How could she kill the one she loved?

***

I've been lost for a while, but I'm back, and I thank you for all you tried to do.

We are connected once again. There was a time we weren't, when I left you. Now I see you, and you see me. Yes, I was the woman you met in the post office and grocery store who looked like me. I knew that would send a tingle into your being, and it did. I'm glad you didn't get her name or where she lived.

I'm the Flutterby who crossed your window. I'm also the red bird you see, chirping, flapping my wings. How great Thou Art.

Now you know I'll never leave you, even though I've passed. The human body is gone, but my being lives on. It's now my job to look after you, watch you live your Journey, visit you in Flutterby wings, and other forms, letting you know you're not alone. Especially when you're depressed, missing me. I know you'll know me because we believed there was more to life after death. And there is.

Geech – Halleluiah … finally I can fly. What a beautiful red color I am. Geech, you called me. I liked the name. You said the name belonged to someone's uncle. Well I'm nobody's uncle yet. I'm only a year old. One thing, I wish you'd buy different bird seed. You see, the sticks get in the way of the sunflower seeds, and I have to spit them on the ground for those big fat doves.

Flutterby – Halleluiah … I'm yellow and black, and fly all over from flower to flower. My long slender legs come in handy, when I land on delicate blue flowers in the back yard.

Fluffeytail … I'm finally Fluffytail of hemlock hall. I can jump from tree to tree. At times even fly from tree to tree. I eat the bird seeds and plant my nuts in holes for next year. Boy, there's a lot of land to plant nuts on. When it comes digging time, I won't be able to find them, because the property's so big.

Thank God, Mr. Tortoise dug a hole under the palmetto bush this year. Fluffytail, Geech, and Flutterby, had a place to stay during the storm. Mr. Tortoise is a mighty nice fellow.

Epilogue

I cared for my dear friend, Carol, for fourteen years, as written, in 'Just a Word' Alzheimer's, but what you've just read is different, some true, some not.

I decided to write this, thinking, I knew Carol's point of view better than anyone, and wanted others to know it. What *she* would say, if able. Being close, connected, I knew what was going on in her mind, even though she couldn't tell me in my words.

I'm sure there are many others who feel the same way. Especially if you've cared for someone with Alzheimer's, or another form of dementia. After a while you take on their voice.

I wrote this story after reading news articles on Alzheimer's and other dementias. Some stories made me sick, knowing what goes on. But others made me happy, knowing in certain states someone with this horrific disease could make their own decision on life or death.

I wish we had a cure for Alzheimer's and dementia, but as of now, 2015, we don't. Some dementia's, if found soon enough can be helped, while most can't. I write letting others know what lay in their path, victim and caregiver.

*****

One of Carol's sayings:

"Think of me as one withdrawn into the dimness, yours still, you mine; remember all the best of our past moments and forget the rest, and so, to where I wait, come gently on."

*****

Other books by Rose Lamatt

Is life One Big Goodbye - 'Homeless Woman's survival story'

Just a Word – Alzheimer's

Connected - 'Online Connection'

Voiceless Cry - 'Panic Attacks and Agoraphobia'

Is Life One Big Goodbye

The cab dropped me off and I stood looking at the building—*Old*. Fanny pack strapped around my waist, and computer bag over my shoulder, I rolled the suitcase behind me, up the steps to my new home. Unable to lower my head, I felt each step before me with my foot and climbed, until I reached the door. I pressed the bell, a buzzer sounded, and I pulled on the knob letting me in. The lobby was small and I saw faces of color. None like mine. Four or five women stood talking, while two children ran around playing hide and seek. I gave my name to the woman behind the desk and she pointed to a couch. "Have a seat," she said.

I did.

I studied the women's faces. They had no expression. Only the children seemed alive. Another woman came from an inner door and said something to the 'desk woman' then walked toward me.

"Ms. Rose?"

I nodded.

"I'm Lena, I spoke to you on the phone yesterday."

"Hello," I said and reached out my hand, the same way I did years ago, meeting golfers for a match at the club. Now I shook this hand, in a Homeless Shelter. "Follow me," she said. "I'll show you your room." I followed, down the long dark hall, to the last door on the right. When she unlocked the door three beds faced us. She walked to the middle one and said, "This is yours, Ms. Rose," then pressed the mattress. "It's nice and soft, feel." I did, and noticed it was harder than the one I had slept in the night before, mine. Opposite the bed, she slid back a door, "This is your closet," she said, then asked, "Is that all you have?" Yes, I said, knowing I didn't want to bring much, I wouldn't be staying long. My main treasures had gone to storage that morning: bed room set, books, family and friends pictures, clothes, and other items that made up ones' life. "Come, I'll show you your bathroom," Lena said, and I followed. She unlocked the door. "This is for Transitional Residents only," she said. (meaning me.) The smell of mold hit me as I looked around: two stalls, two showers, opposite them four sinks under a mirror. A large frosted window took up the end wall. Rust everywhere, paint chipped off walls, floor spotted with paint, same color as the walls, dirty pink. She told me how nice it was, I listened. Back in the hall, she handed me two keys, "Now make sure you don't lose them," she said. "We charge for replacements." I put the keys in my pocket. She shook my hand saying how nice it was that I joined them. I didn't know if *join* was the right word. My other choice was to live on the streets in a cardboard box. I followed her into her office and signed papers. She said I could stay until low-cost housing called, but no longer than twelve months. When done, I left and headed back to my room, using the key given me.

Inside I stood, the door closed behind me. Three beds covered neatly with blue spreads held my sight. I inched closer to the middle one, mine. A fan squeaked above me. The head of the bed rested against cement, not like other walls I'd known: painted ones, wallpapered ones, soft ones. In a daze I unpacked and hung three pairs of slacks, two pairs of jeans, and five blouses in the closet. I placed two pairs of sneakers under the bed. My computer bag, holding my 'savior' lay on the bed. I stood the empty suitcase upright, as a table in the closet for deodorant, toothbrush, toothpaste, and anything else. My pajamas, sweatshirt and sweatpants I folded neatly on the top shelf. It was almost spring, but there was a chill in the air. I prayed I would be gone by summer when I could get my life back in order. It had been out of order too long.

My neck hurting, I lay on the bed hoping for rest, but my thoughts spun round. I prayed low-cost housing would call earlier and surprise me. Six to twelve months' waiting list, the woman on the phone had said. I got up, making sure the keys were in my pocket. I didn't trust my thinking anymore since the neck operation. I was confused and disoriented at times. I walked to the bathroom, unlocked the door, and entered the first stall. I sat, and then realized no toilet paper. Quickly I stood, pulling up my pants, before letting anything out of me. In the lobby I asked the woman behind the desk, "Do you have any toilet paper? There's none in the bathroom."

She pointed to the side counter, "Take a roll. Bring it back when you're done."

No toilet paper in the bathroom? I thought. When done, I returned the roll. The desk woman said, "You need to buy your own."

"Okay," I answered.

Walking out the back door I saw women sitting on a patio smoking. They looked at me and I looked at them, trying to smile, and then followed the sidewalk leading to another building. A sign on the door read Dinner 6 p.m. It was now 5:30, I opened the door. There were couches, chairs, and TV playing a religious station. Double doors led me to the dining room: a large room, long tables, folding chairs, piano off to the side. It was the pictures on the wall facing me that caught my attention. Painted pictures, odd pictures, pictures of faces with black and blue eyes, and the word Jesus painted across them. I looked for a table where I'd eat dinner, maybe in the corner by the window. *Yes*, there. I left by an outside door, and sat on a bench to wait. Children played on the gym in the middle of the sidewalk circle. Three used the slide, while another kicked a ball. They seemed happy, and I wondered if they were? One child, bowlegged, tried to run. He ran, sat, ran, and sat down. He looked around two years old, maybe less. For twenty minutes I watched them, and then saw women and children headed toward the dining room. I looked at my watch, 6:05, and wondered, should I go now? No, I'll wait a little longer. More women and children followed the others, and finally I got up the nerve to join them.

Opening the doors, I heard loud voices and crying children. *Where did they all come from?* I thought. Women sat in chairs along one wall. I stood mesmerized, and someone behind me said, "You need to wait on line, over there. Dinner's not ready." I told the woman to go ahead of me, thinking I could learn from her. The door opened under the Entrance sign and a tall woman in a white coat announced, "Ladies, dinner is served."

In the kitchen, half-way through 'The Line', I realized I'd forgotten utensils, and backed up. Women angrily stared at me as I said, "Excuse me. Excuse me," and grabbed a fork, knife, and spoon. I centered my thoughts on the women in front of me, hoping for direction. Finally, I made it to the Exit door, and found the table off to the side by the window.

Placing the napkin on my lap, and straightening my utensils I looked up. Others stared at me. Was it because they admired my hard-neck-brace? Children probably thought I looked like Hannibal Lecter from *Silence of the Lambs*, or was it because I was White? Only a handful were like me, but younger. I ate turkey, potatoes, bread, and drank strawberry milk, keeping my head down. I ate little due to an upset stomach, and worked the Sudoku puzzle on the back of the milk carton. At least my brain was working. I got it right.

Later, I sat in the shelter's library. A clean room, musty smelling, with pale blue walls and books stacked neatly on shelves almost reaching the ceiling. Three computers sat on a table near the windows and I thought, *maybe I can get online*. I hit the 'on' button, but nothing happened. I tried the other two machines, nothing.

I'd worn my fanny pack since I walked in the front door, afraid someone would steal it. The women were hard looking: piercings everywhere, not only in ears, but lips and eyebrows. I undid the fanny pack clasp and placed it on the table. Two large windows let in light, even though the blinds were closed and the sun was almost down. It wasn't yet hot in central Florida, but come summer, you'd be able to fry an egg on the sidewalk.

I plugged in my 'savior' thinking, *what can I do with it? I can't get online.* All I knew was writing online about Alzheimer's. Then thought, *maybe I'll write a journal. I'll be here a while, besides it'll give me something to do. Yes. A Journal.*

Time had gone quickly, and I had written three pages, my mind off where my body was. I looked at my wrist watch, 10 o'clock, and thought; *I'll have to go sooner or later.*

I walked down the dimly lit hall and used the key given me. Opening the door, the black woman nearest the door looked at me. I thought I saw her smile.

"Hi, I'm Rose," I said, trying to return a smile.

"Hi, I'm Doretta," she said. "That's Linda," and pointed to the white woman lying in bed near the window with ear-buds. "Linda, *Linda*!" Doretta yelled. And the woman lifted her head. She removed the buds, and I repeated my name. "Hi," she said. "Welcome," and buds went back in, doing whatever she was doing before.

From my closet, I got a T-shirt and pajama pants that hung on a side hook.

"Do you work?" Doretta asked.

"No," I said.

Linda and her did, she said, and would be up early. I said, "Okay," and that I'd try to be quiet. I then headed down the hall to change. I didn't change in front of my husband; I surely wasn't going to change in front of strangers.

Opening the bathroom door, a black woman brushed her teeth. She didn't look up and I didn't disturb her. Instead I went in the first stall and peed, wiping with one of the wads of stolen toilet paper from my pocket. I heard the hall door open, then quiet. I was alone. I didn't know these people. They were different than me. I hadn't slept in days, not knowing what lay ahead, and I was scared and tired.

Back in the room, I heard Doretta snore, and TV sounds. I looked at the lighted travel clock, one I had taken to motels, traveling from Florida to Long Island, seeing family and friends, playing golf years ago. At 11:10, I climbed into bed. It was harder than last night's bed. I stared at the turning fan blades above me, and heard its' squeak.

Midnight, Doretta yelled, "Linda, turn the TV lower." No answer. "If you're sleeping, TURN THE DAMN THING OFF!!" Linda jumped up, and hit the button. *Nice*, I thought, *in the middle bed, words flying over me.* I reached for the Rosary beads I'd put under the pillow earlier, and silently mouthed the words, "Our Father who art in heaven ...."